Diabetes *and the* Metabolic Syndrome in Mental Health

Diabetes *and* *the* Metabolic Syndrome in Mental Health

EDITORS

Jennifer A. Rosen, Pharm.D., BCPP

Clinical Pharmacist in Psychiatry
VA Long Beach Healthcare System
Long Beach, California

Donna A. Wirshing, M.D.

Attending Psychiatrist
VA Greater Los Angeles Healthcare System
Los Angeles, California

Wolters Kluwer | Lippincott Williams & Wilkins
Health

Philadelphia • Baltimore • New York • London
Buenos Aires • Hong Kong • Sydney • Tokyo

Acquisitions Editor: Charles W. Mitchell
Managing Editor: Sirkka E. Howes
Project Manager: Jennifer Harper
Manufacturing Coordinator: Kathleen Brown
Marketing Manager: Kimberly Schonberger
Design Coordinator: Steve Druding
Production Services: International Typesetting and Composition

© 2008 by LIPPINCOTT WILLIAMS & WILKINS, a WOLTERS KLUWER business
530 Walnut Street
Philadelphia, PA 19106 USA
LWW.com

Printed in the USA

Library of Congress Cataloging-in-Publication Data

Diabetes and the metabolic syndrome in mental health / editors, Jennifer A. Rosen, Donna A. Wirshing.
  p. ; cm.
  Includes bibliographical references and index.
  ISBN-13: 978-0-7817-8270-8 (alk. paper)
  ISBN-10: 0-7817-8270-8 (alk. paper)
 1. Diabetes.   2. Metabolism—Disorders.   3. Mentally ill—Diseases.
I. Rosen, Jennifer A.   II. Wirshing, Donna.
  [DNLM: 1. Diabetes Mellitus.   2. Mentally Ill Persons.   WK 810 D53752537
2008]
  RC660.D4493 2008
  616.4'62—dc22

                                        2007050598

   Care has been taken to confirm the accuracy of the information presented and to describe generally accepted practices. However, the authors, editors, and publisher are not responsible for errors or omissions or for any consequences from application of the information in this book and make no warranty, expressed or implied, with respect to the currency, completeness, or accuracy of the contents of the publication. Application of the information in a particular situation remains the professional responsibility of the practitioner.
   The authors, editors, and publisher have exerted every effort to ensure that drug selection and dosage set forth in this text are in accordance with current recommendations and practice at the time of publication. However, in view of ongoing research, changes in government regulations, and the constant flow of information relating to drug therapy and drug reactions, the reader is urged to check the package insert for each drug for any change in indications and dosage and for added warnings and precautions. This is particularly important when the recommended agent is a new or infrequently employed drug.
   Some drugs and medical devices presented in the publication have Food and Drug Administration (FDA) clearance for limited use in restricted research settings. It is the responsibility of the health care provider to ascertain the FDA status of each drug or device planned for use in their clinical practice.

To purchase additional copies of this book, call our customer service department at (800) 638-3030 or fax orders to (301) 223-2320. International customers should call (301) 223-2300.

Visit Lippincott Williams & Wilkins on the Internet: at LWW.com. Lippincott Williams & Wilkins customer service representatives are available from 8:30 am to 6 pm, EST.

                                        10 9 8 7 6 5 4 3 2 1

*We would like to dedicate this book
to our patients, who serve as
our daily inspiration.*

CONTENTS

PREFACE

Over the years, my patients have been my greatest teachers. This book is dedicated to these great teachers. When I think of the challenges of living with mental illness and diabetes, I think of Michael, my first teacher. Michael was one of my very first patients on an inpatient psychiatric ward. He was a man with schizophrenia and very advanced diabetes. I first met him in the kidney dialysis unit of our hospital, where I was called to see him because he was terribly depressed, suicidal, and refusing treatment. The diabetes had also caused him to become blind and to lose one of his legs. He was wheelchair-bound in a dark, confusing world. After I spoke with him, he resolved to allow himself to undergo dialysis. Michael taught me about the extraordinary challenge of facing both life-threatening psychiatric and medical conditions. Here, I became immersed in the challenge the medical and psychiatric teams to provide uncomfortable, yet necessary treatment—dialysis to a blind man whose mind was ravaged by paranoia and auditory hallucinations.

I thought Michael's resolve to remain in treatment was quite extraordinary. I was equally impressed by the care of the nurses and physicians in the dialysis unit who humored him through these difficult sessions. With the excellent collaborative care he received, Michael lived for 10 years following my first meeting with him, but I often wondered, at what cost, and with what quality of life? What could have been done differently to prevent this series of events that resulted in such discomfort and cost to Michael, to his family, and to society?

The epidemic of diabetes has affected the entire United States and it has not excluded the many patients with severe mental illness. This epidemic is costing the nation billions of dollars in direct and indirect costs, resulting in a huge public health crisis.

It is estimated that 7% of the people in the United States have diabetes, and that another 7% are undiagnosed. In 2005, 1.5 million new cases of diabetes were diagnosed in people over 20 years of age. The epidemic in children is even more of a concern. It is estimated that 1 in 3 children born in the year 2000 will develop diabetes, and that one in two Hispanic children born that year will develop diabetes.[1]

In this book, we will explore the prevalence of diabetes in patients with mental illnesses and the role of cortisol in relation to diabetes. We will discuss the costs related to the treatment of diabetes and its comorbidities, and the legal ramifications doctors must consider when prescribing medications that may potentially worsen or precipitate new-onset diabetes. We will also review the relationship between various pharmacotherapies used to treat psychiatric disorders that may impact and actually cause new-onset diabetes and other metabolic disorders, either directly or indirectly, by contributing to obesity.

Our research group was among the first in the field to identify a possible link between the development of obesity, diabetes, and other metabolic derangements (e.g., lipid abnormalities) and the use of newer, second-generation antipsychotic medications. We will review the scientific literature on this particular subject, as well as discuss the association between antidepressants and mood stabilizers, and diabetes.

Finally, we will elaborate on the latest research in regards to the prevention and management of obesity and diabetes in patients with severe mental illness. We provide the reader with resources to help patients who suffer from these comorbidities.

We hope that this will be a useful resource for clinicians treating mentally ill patients with diabetes, so that clinicians can learn more about diabetes, as well as about the link between mental illness, its pharmacotherapies, and diabetes. Ultimately, we hope that this book will serve as a tool for prevention of diabetes and the devastating incapacitation of blindness, kidney failure, and limb loss that my very first patient with schizophrenia endured. We do not expect a psychiatrist to become an endocrinologist, or an endocrinologist to become a psychiatrist, but we do hope that this book can help with the collaborative process needed to provide comprehensive medical care to patients like Michael, challenged by both diseases.

1. Facing the diabetes epidemic-mandatory reporting of glycosylated hemoglobin values in New York City. *New Engl Journal Med.* 2006;354(6): 545–548.

Jennifer A. Rosen, Pharm.D., BCPP
Donna A. Wirshing M.D.

CONTRIBUTORS

Jacob S. Ballon, M.D.
Resident, Department of Psychiatry, Stanford University, Stanford, California

Shahla S. Cano, R.D., C.D.E.
Clinical Nutrition Educator, Health Education/Medicine, Kaiser Permanente, Deer Valley, California

Gale Z. Feldman, M.P.H.
Principal Consultant, Feldman, Milliken & Associates—Consulting in Community Health, Santa Monica, California

Jamie W. Fernandez, M.D.
Resident, Department of Psychiatry, Stanford University; Resident, Department of Psychiatry and Behavioral Sciences, Stanford University Hospital and Clinics, Stanford, California

Cara F. Adamson Greene, Pharm.D.
Research Health Science Specialist, Department of Psychiatry, VA Greater Los Angeles Healthcare System, Los Angeles, California

Arlene E. Johns, M.P.H., R.D., C.N.S.D.
Clinical Dietician, Food and Nutrition Services, Kaiser Permanente Los Angeles Medical Center, Los Angeles, California

Vasanthi L. Narayan, M.D.
Clinical Fellow in Endocrinology, UCLA-VA Greater Los Angeles Healthcare System, Los Angeles, California

Jennifer A. Rosen, Pharm. D. BCPP
Clinical Pharmacist in Psychiatry, Department of Pharmacy, VA Long Beach Healthcare System, Long Beach, California

Eda Vesterman, M.S.
Chef/Dietitian, Culinary Department, The Art Institute of California, Orange County, California; Dietitian, Research Department, VAGLHS/UCLA, Los Angeles, California

Jane E. Weinreb, M.D.
Assistant Professor of Clinical Medicine, David Geffen School of Medicine at UCLA; Chief, Diabetes Program, VA Greater Los Angeles Healthcare System at West LA, Los Angeles, California

Jeremy M. Wilkinson, M.D.
Resident, Department of Psychiatry, San Mateo Medical Center, San Mateo, California

Diabetes *and the* Metabolic Syndrome in Mental Health

CHAPTER 1

Diabetes and Mental Health

Jacob S. Ballon and Jamie W. Fernandez

Overview of the Problem

Major depression, bipolar disorder, and schizophrenia are severe mental illnesses that affect the lives of those who suffer from them in multiple ways. Social functioning, occupational functioning, and overall quality of life are all core symptoms of psychiatric illness. However, other more subtle issues can influence the lives of those with severe mental illness. Those with mental illness are at higher risk and are more likely to suffer the severe consequences of comorbid medical illness. Adherence to treatment is often more difficult, and other factors such as psychoneuroendocrine interactions may complicate already problematic treatments. Additionally, psychiatric medications themselves often have severe side effects and can interact with other medications, rendering treatment of the mental illness more complicated.

Diabetes is one example of a comorbid medical illness that is seen at a higher rate in people with mental illness. Complications of diabetes are severe, including blindness, renal failure, neuropathy, impaired immune function, amputation, and cardiovascular disease. Acute mismanagement of blood glucose can lead to hypoglycemia or, if treatment is neglected, to severe hyperglycemia and coma or death. In this chapter, the severity of the problem of diabetes in depression, schizophrenia, and bipolar disorder will be discussed.

The Relationship Between Cortisol, Stress, and Diabetes

Cortisol is a steroid hormone that has long been associated with stress, either physiological or psychological. As stress mounts, corticotropin-releasing hormone is released from the hypothalamus, which leads to release of adrenocorticotropic hormone from the pituitary and causes the adrenal gland to release glucocorticoids, including cortisol. Concurrently, stimulation at the locus ceruleus leads to further adrenergic output. Increased adrenergic output results in hyperarousal, improvement in selective attention, and decreased neurovegetative behaviors. The so-called "fight or flight" response allows a person to physiologically respond quickly to a stressful situation. In the short-term, the stress response can be beneficial; however, a prolonged or chronic state of stress has been shown to be associated with higher morbidity.[1]

Diabetes is a disorder of the endocrine system in which dysregulation of insulin and glucagon result in abnormal levels of blood sugar. Although several pathways lead to diabetes, the final common pathway yields an elevation of blood glucose. Cortisol plays a role in regulation of body fat distribution and can lead to increased lipolysis when glucose levels become substantial or in times of diabetic ketoacidosis. This can result in overburdening of the oxidative pathways and lead to complications of hepatic steatosis and hypertriglyceridemia. Intra-abdominal fat deposits have been shown to have higher insulin resistance than more peripheral fat. Additionally, because they are more prone to lipolysis and thus circulating as free fatty acids, they distribute aspects of insulin resistance to the liver and peripheral muscles. The impact of cortisol on the distribution of body fat, particularly in people prone to higher levels of cortisol, can lead to worsening of both mood and glucose regulation.[2]

Psychoneuroendocrine theories stem initially from observations of disease states related to glucocorticoid dysfunction. In Cushing's disease, a state of pathological hypercortisolemia, more than 50% of patients have a comorbid depressive state. On the opposite side of the cortisol spectrum, in Addison's disease, a state of adrenal insufficiency and glucocorticoid depletion, apathy, insomnia, and social withdrawal frequently accompany the characteristic fatigue and muscle weakness. In both conditions, normalization of hormone levels leads to symptom relief.[3] Additionally, treatment with exogenous steroids for inflammatory disorders or for illicit purposes often has profound mood complications, and suicides and uncontrollable rage have been linked to steroid use.[4]

Depression: Given the above mentioned relationship that cortisol has with stress, mood, and metabolism, it was reasonable to hypothesize that cortisol could be a unifying causative factor in the increased rate of diabetes in depression. A recent Italian study showed that older adults with depression and hypercortisolemia had a synergistically greater risk of a metabolic syndrome compared with other older adults.[5]

Hypercortisolemic states have also long been linked to psychotic major depression (PMD).[6] In rats, it has been shown that exogenous dexamethasone leads to increased dopamine in the nucleus accumbens, which is also associated with psychotic symptoms.[7] Mifepristone, a glucocorticoid receptor antagonist (better known for its effects on progesterone that allow it to be used as an abortifacient), has been shown to work quickly to help treat the symptoms of PMD. In an industry-sponsored, placebo-controlled trial of mifepristone, when the drug was used in a 7-day course, it showed significant benefits for psychotic symptoms at 7 days and persistent 56 days later. Interestingly, mifepristone had no beneficial effect on depressive symptoms, and both the placebo group and mifepristone groups had similar rates of subsequent antidepressant, antipsychotic, and electroconvulsive therapy use at 7 days, which persisted for 56 days. Because this was an inpatient study that required daily assessments, there was a higher placebo response than in typical PMD studies, and this may have obscured antidepressant benefits, according to the authors.[8] In small open-label and placebo-crossover trials, mifepristone has been previously shown to be beneficial in the treatment of PMD.[9,10]

Racial differences are apparent in the impact of cortisol on glucose in depressed patients. In a large study of veterans, there was a greater magnitude of glucose dysregulation in African Americans compared with whites, with higher levels of hypothalamic-pituitary-adrenal (HPA) axis activity seen as a direct mediator of that effect.[11]

Although most of the research has focused on dysregulation of cortisol and the HPA axis, others argue that insulin and hyperglycemia may have a direct impact on the brain and that hypercortisolemia may be a more downstream effect of that dysregulation. Thus, insulin may be the primary factor linking diabetes and depression, with cortisol a secondary contributor.[12]

According to the World Health Organization, unipolar major depression is considered the greatest cause of disability in terms of disability-adjusted life years in the world.[13] People with depression are known to have an increased rate of comorbid medical and psychiatric illnesses. Multiple studies have shown that depression likewise can also be a harbinger of diabetes.[14,15] Additionally, rates of depression are often higher in people with diabetes. Often the two illnesses share similar characteristic symptoms, such as apathy and decreased energy at onset. The stress hormone cortisol is typically elevated in depression. As cortisol levels change, psychoneuroendocrinological changes disrupt hormonal regulation further downstream and can lead to changes in mood as well as glucose homeostasis.

Depression rates have been studied and are increased in type 1 and type 2 diabetes. In a meta-analysis, Barnard et al. reviewed 14 trials in which patients with type 1 diabetes were surveyed for rates of depression.[16] When these researchers looked at all the trials, they found that subjects with type 1 diabetes had a 12.0% rate of depression compared with a rate of 3.4% in those without diabetes. In noncontrolled trials, they found an even higher rate of depression in patients with type 1 diabetes (13.4%). However, despite these overall findings, in trials that were considered of an adequate design, and with a substantially rigorous depression screening method (i.e., use of structured clinical interview rather than patient reported surveys), the rates were not statistically significantly increased (odds ratio [OR] = 2.36, 95% confidence interval [CI] = 0.69–5.4) but had such substantial variation that it was not sufficient to draw a conclusion regarding type 1 diabetes.

In an international study, patients with type 1 diabetes were also examined by Lloyd et al.[17] Looking at sites in Pittsburgh, Pennsylvania (n = 131) and Birmingham, England (n = 77), patients were rated on the Beck

Depression Inventory and the Beck Anxiety Inventory. Patients with moderate to severe anxiety or depression were grouped together. The British group was noted to have a higher rate of moderate-severe anxiety (17% vs. 5%, p = 0.0002) compared with the group in Pittsburgh. Despite finding that patients with higher anxiety scores were correlated with depressed mood and decreased physical activity, there was only a slight difference between the groups in the rate of moderate to severe depression (9% England, 7% Pittsburgh, p = 0.6337). In contrast to other studies, which have suggested that people with depression have poorer self-care, self-care was not generally noted to differ among the groups in this study. The only exception was that in British women with anxiety, there was a noted increase in the frequency of blood glucose monitoring.[17]

When it comes to rates of depression, type 2 diabetes has been studied more extensively than type 1 diabetes. Anderson et al. compiled a large meta-analysis, looking at 42 studies involving more than 21,000 subjects to assess rates of depression among patients with type 1 versus type 2 diabetes mellitus.[18] Regardless of how depression was measured, type 1 diabetes was associated with lower rates of depression than type 2 diabetes. Patients' self-reported scores revealed higher rates of depression than structured clinical interviews, and women with diabetes had higher rates of depression than men, although in a similar fashion to the population without diabetes. Depression was significantly increased in both type 1 and type 2 diabetes, with increased ORs for subjects with type 1 (OR = 2.9, 95% CI 1.6 –5.5, χ^2 = 12.8, p = 0.0003) and type 2 disease (OR = 2.9, 95% CI 2.3–3.7, χ^2 = 84.3, p = 0.0001) compared with controls. Overall, with multiple factors controlled for, the risk of depression in people with diabetes was approximately twofold.

In another large meta-analysis, Ali et al. looked at more than 51,000 subjects in ten different studies to assess rates of depression in type 2 diabetes mellitus.[19] The results demonstrate that rates of diabetes are increased in both men and women, and like the other studies, the rates are increased for women compared with men. However, the OR for comorbid depression among the diabetic patients studied was higher for men than for women, indicating that although women with diabetes have an overall increased prevalence of depression (23.8 vs. 12.8%, p < 0.0001), men with diabetes have an increased risk of developing depression (men: OR = 1.9, 95% CI 1.7–2.1 vs. women: OR = 1.3, 95% CI 1.2–1.4).

In the elderly (age 70–79, n = 3,075), Maraldi et al. recently reported an increase in depression among those with type 2 diabetes over an average of 6 years follow-up.[20] Additionally, those with worse glycemic control showed an increased frequency of depressive symptoms. Even without meeting the diagnostic threshold for major depressive disorder, in the elderly, the presence of diabetes contributed to an increased risk of recurrent depressed mood. Depression was likewise also independently associated with decreased cognitive function, slowed gait speed, and obesity.

In children, depression has been evaluated primarily in the type 1 population. Although the prevalence of type 2 diabetes in children is increasing, the literature focuses more on type 1 disease. The treatment of type 1 diabetes can be traumatic in itself, with frequent finger sticks to measure blood glucose and frequent subcutaneous insulin injections to manage glucose levels. Research has shown that youths 12–17 years of age with type 1 diabetes had double the risk of depression compared with a teenage population without diabetes.[21] This amounted to nearly 15% of children meeting the criteria for depression. These data also highlight the importance of family support and healthy family dynamics in diabetes treatment outcomes and overall mood outcomes in the adolescent population. Disagreements in subjective assessments of the mood of children with diabetes often have led to disagreements in other aspects of their care, and thus multidisciplinary teams can prove helpful in aligning the needs of the children and expectations of parents.

To this point, depression has only been discussed as being more prevalent among patients with diabetes. However, few studies look to identify if depression is a risk factor for diabetes or vice versa. Knol et al. performed a meta-analysis in an attempt to answer this question.[22] Pooling data from nine studies, these researchers found that people with depression carried a nearly 40% risk of developing diabetes. Although they caution that reverse causality could be a potential bias (namely, people with presymptomatic diabetes may show signs of depression prior to the onset of meeting the diagnostic threshold for diabetes), other studies that have excluded such subjects show generally the same results.

Schizophrenia: The relationship between schizophrenia and diabetes goes back well over 100 years. As has been mentioned earlier with respect to depression, there are also psychoneuroendocrine factors that appear to link diabetes and schizophrenia. Early studies in both humans and cats noted an increase in glucosuria under times of stress. These effects were noticed to be magnified in people with schizophrenia when they were admitted to the hospital in the early 1900s, particularly if they were in an agitated rather than an apathetic state.[23] These findings were replicated several times prior to the advent of antipsychotic medication.[24] In a study of veterans with schizophrenia, nearly 70% of patients showed abnormal glucose values on a 1-hour glucose tolerance test compared with 30% in a control group without schizophrenia. Although no correlation was drawn in this study with adrenaline secretion, some subtypes noted on Rorschach testing appeared more likely to have the abnormal glucose results.[25]

In the first few decades of the 1900s, prior to the advent of antipsychotic medication, psychiatrists experimented with various treatment options, including electroconvulsive therapy. With the discovery of insulin in 1910s, its use was pioneered by Sakel in Austria with the development of insulin coma therapy, which reached prominence by the late 1930s. The theory related to the purported neurotransmitter effect of insulin and its relation to psychosis. Although the treatment was effective for many patients, evidence was primarily anecdotal and not subjected to the rigors of controlled trials, as it would be today. Ultimately, the procedure was difficult and often dangerous, thus easily giving way to antipsychotic medications in the early 1950s.[26]

Upon the discovery of chlorpromazine, a prevailing theory was that the increased prevalence of diabetes among patients with schizophrenia taking antipsychotic medication resulted from an unmasking of a previously elevated risk of diabetes inherent schizophrenics.[27] Recently, this problem has been exacerbated by the contribution of second-generation antipsychotic medications toward increasing the risk of insulin resistance, metabolic syndrome, and diabetes. A further discussion of this aspect of schizophrenia and diabetes will follow in later chapters.

Although type 2 diabetes mellitus typically comes to mind when one thinks of schizophrenia and diabetes, it is important not to overlook the comorbidity of type 1 diabetes and schizophrenia. Type 1 diabetes requires careful and consistent monitoring of blood glucose, and the cognitive disorganization and confusion that can result from exacerbations of psychosis can be disruptive and especially dangerous in these patients. Fortunately, epidemiological research has demonstrated an inverse relationship between schizophrenia and type 1 diabetes. In a study from Finland, researchers collected data from every patient identified from a national registry with type 1 diabetes from 1950 through 1959. Although the rate of schizophrenia was 0.56 per 10,000 person-years in the group without type 1 diabetes, for people with the diabetes, there was a rate of schizophrenia of 0.21 per 10,000 person-years. It is necessary to consider that ascertainment bias can always be a confounding factor with these types of results (i.e., how people are identified as having either disorder is dependent on their contact with the national health registry).

Interestingly, although neither disease, schizophrenia or diabetes, is fully explained on the basis of current genetic findings, there are some areas of overlap in genetic risk factors (i.e., HLA subtype A24 and DQB1*0602). Ultimately, the relationship between these two illnesses remains elusive, with theories related to the risk of harm from maternal infection, genetic disequilibrium, or environmental factors leading to the decreased risk of schizophrenia in patients with type 1 diabetes.[28]

Although patients with type 1 diabetes may have a decreased risk of schizophrenia, the same is not true for those with type 2 diabetes. Type 2 diabetes, which is associated with central adiposity, has often been considered linked to schizophrenia, either by the mechanisms discussed above or secondary to lifestyle factors (poor diet, lack of exercise) related to the negative symptoms of schizophrenia itself.

Rates of diabetes in schizophrenia have increased sharply over the years as well. Although rates of type 2 diabetes have increased in the general population over the last generation and continue to increase substantially, the rates in schizophrenia have also increased.[29] The rate of diabetes in schizophrenia is often seen to be approximately two times that of the general population.[30]

As will be discussed later, much has been attributed to the second-generation antipsychotic medications. In an epidemiological look at cohorts of patients discharged from the hospital in the 1980s (before the advent of second-generation antipsychotics), versus those from the early 1990s (at the release of the first of the second-generation antipsychotics), versus those in the early part of this century (reflecting an increase use of the second-generation antipsychotics), the rates of diabetes was seen to have increased 0.7% per year from 1996 to 2001. Groups considered at highest risk for diabetes were African Americans and middle-aged adults.[31]

Even in the era of second-generation antipsychotic medications, however, the rate of diabetes in newly diagnosed cases of schizophrenia is still increased over that of the general population. Looking at cases prospectively using a glucose tolerance test, De Hert et al. have shown an increased risk of diabetes even in people new to the diagnosis and naïve to medication. Although the risk continues to increase throughout the duration of illness, secondary factors such as medication side effects may play a more prominent role. In this study, the risk of diabetes was more than 19% in middle-aged patients who had been treated for many years, compared with nearly 2% in newly diagnosed patients, and risk was shown to increase linearly with age.[32] These data argue strongly that diabetes needs to be considered in all patients with schizophrenia, from the time of diagnosis, throughout the person's lifetime.[33]

The impact of diabetes can be devastating. As the maintenance of a diabetic regimen can at times be difficult, the long-term consequences of hyperglycemia plague patients with schizophrenia. Rates of heart disease and the metabolic syndrome are increased and are the leading cause of premature mortality for people with schizophrenia.[34] Blindness, infection, renal dysfunction, and neuropathy are all sources of significant morbidity related to chronic hyperglycemia. Problems with medication adherence and commitment to preventive regimens (i.e., proper foot care, preventive ophthalmological examinations, and close follow-up with primary care) ultimately may make treating comorbid diabetes and schizophrenia more difficult. Additionally, because rates of smoking are known to be higher among people with schizophrenia, the risk of cardiovascular disease becomes even greater.[35]

Bipolar Illness: Data supporting an association between abnormalities in glucose homeostasis and bipolar disorder has been documented for nearly 100 years. As early as 1919, studies were performed that supported a role for abnormal carbohydrate metabolism in mental disorders.[23,36–38] In an early study by Gildea et al., abnormal glucose tolerance tests after oral administration of dextrose in manic-depressive patients were reported. In this study of 30 patients from 18 to 64 years of age, 20% had an abnormal decline in blood sugar following oral but not intravenous dextrose.[39] Similarly, two studies conducted by Van der Velde and Gordon revealed higher frequencies of abnormal glucose tolerance in manic patients as compared to patients with schizophrenia. In the first study, hospitalized patients with bipolar disorder (N = 42) were compared to an equal number of hospitalized, age-matched patients with schizophrenia. Glucose tolerance test values were taken fasting, and at 30 minutes, 1 hour, and 2 hours after ingesting 75 g of glucose. Fifty percent of patients with bipolar disorder older than 40 years of age (16/32) had an abnormal response (values >600 mg/dL) and 20% (6/32) of patients with schizophrenia had a hyperglycemic response.[40]

Increased rates of comorbid diabetes in patients with bipolar disorder have also previously been shown by Lilliker in two retrospective chart reviews. In a study of 203 manic-depressive patients (defined by the *Diagnostic and Statistical Manual of Mental Disorders,* second edition [DSM II]), 10% (20) had been diagnosed with diabetes mellitus. Patients older than 45 years of age had a prevalence of diabetes of 18% (women) and 6% (men), whereas those patients older than 65 years of age had a prevalence of 23% (women) and 16% (men).[41] Similarly, of 4,508 patients from 18 to 79 years of age discharged between 1973 and 1978, 12.4% of manic-depressive patients were on a diabetic diet compared with 3.3% of schizophrenics and 2.8% overall.[41,42] Although the exact etiology of the relationship between diabetes and bipolar disorder remains unknown, hypotheses have included a genetic relationship between the two disorders, a causal relationship in which diabetic vascular lesions contribute to mood instability, overactivity of the HPA axis and cortisol dysregulation as part of chronic stress resulting from both the manic and depressive phases of the illness, and psychotropic medications.[43–46]

Additional support for this association has been provided by cross-sectional studies of bipolar patients which reveal a high prevalence of type 2 diabetes and poorer subsequent psychiatric outcomes. In one such study, the prevalence of diabetes mellitus was significantly higher in hospitalized bipolar patients than in the general population. This study of 345 hospitalized patients 20 to 74 years of age who met DSM III-R criteria for bipolar disorder (manic or mixed subtype) revealed a prevalence of diabetes of 9.9%, compared with 3.4% in the general population. Interestingly, this study also showed that although the patient's age at first hospitalization and the duration of the psychiatric disorder was generally equivalent for both groups, patients with comorbid diabetes had significantly more lifetime psychiatric hospitalizations.[46] Thus, one can hypothesize that, for bipolar patients, a diagnosis of comorbid diabetes suggests more severe psychiatric pathology, the result of significant dysregulation of a shared pathway.

Kilbourne et al. designed a cross-sectional study to examine the prevalence of general medical conditions in 4,310 patients diagnosed with bipolar disorder in the Veterans Administration (VA) in 2001. The most prevalent conditions among patients with bipolar disorder were compared with the prevalence of each condition in the national database of the VA patient population. Diabetes ranked among these conditions with a prevalence of 17%, and when compared with national data, the prevalence of diabetes was higher in the bipolar cohort than in the national cohort (17.2% vs. 15.6%, $p = 0.0035$).[47]

Because much of the compiled data have included patients treated with psychotropic medications known to promote hyperglycemia, it is tempting to attribute the increased prevalence of type 2 diabetes in patients with bipolar disorder to adverse effects from these medications. There are, however, studies that support an intrinsic relationship between abnormal glucose metabolism and psychiatric disorders. In a retrospective study by Regenold et al., the medical records of 243 inpatients 50 to 74 years of age with diagnoses of either major depression, bipolar I disorder (N = 53), schizoaffective disorder, schizophrenia, or dementia were reviewed for psychiatric and type 2 diabetes mellitus diagnoses. Medications, body mass index (BMI), age, gender, and race were also recorded. The prevalence of diabetes was compared to age, race, and gender-matched rates in the U.S. general population. The overall prevalence of type 2 diabetes for the bipolar disorder subset was 26% (N = 14), compared with 13% in matched controls. Although these patients tended to have a higher BMI, they had not received more treatment with psychotropic medications. A logistic regression analysis model constructed based on the data collected revealed BMI (Wald χ^2 = 9.97, degrees of freedom [DF] = 1, p = 0.002) and psychiatric diagnosis (Wald χ^2 = 11.3, DF = 4, p = 0.02) to be the only independent and statistically significant predictors of a diagnosis of diabetes. All other variables, including the use of potentially hyperglycemic-causing medications, phenothiazines, clozapine, and olanzapine, did not improve prediction of a diabetes diagnosis.[48]

Similarly, a retrospective study looking at patients from the Maritime Bipolar Registry (N = 222), 15 to 82 years of age, with diagnoses of bipolar disorder I (n = 151), bipolar disorder II (n = 65), and bipolar disorder not otherwise specified (N = 6), revealed a more severe course of illness and worse outcomes for patients with comorbid diabetes, irrespective of antipsychotic medication use. In this study, the prevalence of diabetes was 11.7%. Such patients were more likely to be older (53 +/− 10 vs. 43 +/− 12), were chronically ill, rapid cycling, and had lower global assessment of functioning (GAF) scores. In addition, this study revealed that bipolar patients with diabetes had more long-term disability, higher BMI (34 +/− 6 vs. 29 +/− 6), and higher rates of hypertension.[49]

Evidence continues to emerge that suggests that the prevalence of type 2 diabetes mellitus may be increased several times in bipolar disorder. As with obesity and cardiovascular disease, comorbid diabetes in patients with bipolar disorder is also associated with a more severe course of illness, a decrease in GAF, and other medical comorbidities.[50] Thus, it is important to carefully screen and monitor patients with bipolar disorder for diabetes to promote an improved prognosis for this patient population.

Polycystic ovary syndrome (PCOS), a common syndrome characterized by ovulatory dysfunction and hyperandrogenism, has also been shown to be prevalent in patients with manic-depressive illness.[51] The diagnosis of PCOS has lifelong implications, including an increased risk of metabolic syndrome, type 2 diabetes mellitus, and cardiovascular disease.[52] According to the Rotterdam-European Society of Human Reproduction (ESHRE)/American

Society for Reproductive Medicine (ASRAM)–sponsored PCOS consensus workshop group, PCOS is a syndrome of ovarian dysfunction characterized by an association between hyperandrogenism and menstrual irregularities. The typical endocrine profile is increased luteinizing hormone (LH) and testosterone, and low to normal follicle-simulating hormone (FSH). PCOS affects approximately 5% of reproductive age women in the general population.[53,54] Hyperandrogen production by the ovaries in PCOS results from dysregulation of the hypothalamic-pituitary-gonadal axis. More frequent LH pulses lead to increased androgen synthesis by the ovarian theca cells. In patients with PCOS, increased LH pulse frequency is the downstream result of increased gonadotropin-releasing hormone pulses, which is the result of intrinsic abnormalities in hypothalamic production of this hormone. Consequently, the production of LH is favored over FSH in these patients.[55]

It is well known that valproic acid is useful in patients with bipolar disorder and PCOS is one recognized possible side effect of valproic acid. However, some studies suggest higher rates of menstrual irregularities and PCOS in women with bipolar disorder, which is independent of valproic acid treatment when compared to the general population. However, data addressing the relationship between bipolar disorder and PCOS are limited and the existence of a relationship in patients not treated with valproic acid is controversial. Much of the data in this area come from studies of women with epilepsy, which have shown that there is an association between valproate use and characteristic features of PCOS.[56] A study of 140 women with bipolar disorder revealed that nearly 50% taking valproate had menstrual abnormalities and hyperandrogenism and 41% had PCOS. Of those that were not receiving valproate, only 13% has menstrual abnormalities.[57]

Klipstein et al. analyzed women with PCOS for an intrinsic association between PCOS and bipolar disorder independent of pharmacotherapy. In a study of 78 women with PCOS screened for bipolar disorder using the Mood Disorders Questionnaire (MDQ; a validated self-assessment screen for bipolar disorder), 28% had either a previous bipolar diagnosis or met MDQ criteria for bipolar screening positivity. Nearly all (97%) of these women had no history of valproate exposure prior to the diagnosis of PCOS, again eluding to a link between PCOS and bipolar screen positivity and consistent with a potential shared hypothalamic-pituitary-gonadal axis abnormality.[58] Another study found high rates of menstrual abnormalities in women that predated a diagnosis of and treatment for bipolar disorder. In this study of 80 women, 65% reported menstrual abnormalities and 50% reported one or more menstrual abnormalities that preceded a diagnosis of bipolar disorder and treatment.[59]

Nearly 40% of women with PCOS develop impaired glucose tolerance or overt type 2 diabetes, a finding that has been consistent across several geographic areas and ethnic groups. Likewise, women with PCOS are more likely than normal controls to have insulin resistance.[52] The prevalence of PCOS in patients with bipolar disorder suggests overlap in abnormalities of hypothalamic-pituitary function and its downstream effects. Abnormalities of the

hypothalamic-pituitary-gonadal axis, as well as high rates of menstrual disturbances, can occur in patients with bipolar disorder.[60] In fact, one study showed
that both occurred in the context of obesity and irrespective of medication used.[61]

Freeman and Gelenberg conducted a literature search of MEDLINE
journals from 1965 to the present in order to review the presentation, clinical course, and treatment considerations of bipolar disorder in women.[62]
Treatment-related issues included PCOS, weight gain and obesity, and medication interactions with oral contraceptives. Their results showed that
women with bipolar disorder might be more vulnerable to mood episodes in
the context of reproductive events. However, in PCOS, the researchers
believed that more data are needed to guide treatment decisions.[62] This
study, in combination with the paucity of existing data, points to the urgent
need for further data in these areas to deliver care that is more suitable to
women with bipolar disorder.

As many as 30% to 40% of women with PCOS have insulin resistance by
their fourth decade and approximately 10% will develop diabetes, emphasiz-
ing the importance of glucose monitoring and close follow-up in these
patients.[63,64] In patients who have received both a diagnosis of bipolar disorder and PCOS this is particularly relevant, given the high prevalence of type
2 diabetes within both populations.

Conclusion

Although the links are not fully understood, there is a relationship between
the endocrine system and the neuropsychiatric sequelae of schizophrenia and
bipolar disorder. Unfortunately, this predisposition for diabetes is often worsened by treatment with antipsychotic medication. In addition to the medical
complications, there is a substantial cost burden shouldered by patients and
the medical system. Increased hospitalizations, poor medication adherence
and decreased commitment to preventive regimens all highlight the great
importance for clinicians to be aware of and aggressive in their treatment of
comorbid diabetes.

References

1. Dimsdale JE, Irwin M, Keefe FJ, et al. Stress and psychiatry. In: Sadock BJ, Sadock
   VA, eds. *Kaplan & Sadock's comprehensive textbook of psychiatry.* 8th ed.
   Philadelphia PA. Williams & Wilkins; 2005:2188–2194.
2. Sherwin R. Diabetes mellitus. In: Goldman L, Ausiello D, eds. *Cecil textbook of
   medicine.* 22nd ed. WB Saunders, Philadelphia PA; 2004: Chapter 242.
3. Thase ME. Mood disorders: neurobiology. In: Sadock BJ, Sadock VA, eds. *Kaplan
   & Sadock's comprehensive textbook of psychiatry.* 8th ed. 2005:1595–1603.
4. Thiblin I, Runeson B, Rajs J. Anabolic androgenic steroids and suicide. *Ann Clin
   Psychiatry.* 1999;11(4):223–241.
5. Vogelzangs N, Suthers K, Ferrucci L, et al. Hypercortisolemic depression is associated
   with the metabolic syndrome in late-life. *Psychoneuroendocrinology.* 2007;32(2):151–159.

6. Schatzberg AF, Rothschild AJ, Langlais PJ, et al. A corticosteroid/dopamine hypothesis for psychotic depression and related states. *J Psych Res.* 1985;19(1):57–64.

7. Rothschild AJ, Langlais PJ, Schatzberg AF, et al. The effects of a single acute dose of dexamethasone on monoamine and metabolite levels in rat brain. *Life Sci.* 1985;36(26):2491–2501.

8. DeBattista C, Belanoff J, Glass S, et al. Mifepristone versus placebo in the treatment of psychosis in patients with psychotic major depression. *Biol. Psychiatry.* 2006;60(12):1343–1349.

9. Belanoff JK, Rothschild AJ, Cassidy F, et al. An open label trial of C-1073 (mifepristone) for psychotic major depression. *Biol. Psychiatry.* 2002;52(5):386–392.

10. Belanoff JK, Flores BH, Kalezhan M, et al. Rapid reversal of psychotic depression using mifepristone. *J Clin Psychopharmacol.* 2001;21(5):516–521.

11. Boyle SH, Surwit RS, Georgiades A, et al. Depressive symptoms, race and glucose concentrations: the role of cortisol as mediator. *Diabetes Care.* 2007; 30:2484–2488.

12. Castillo Q, Herrera G, Pérez O. Insulin-cortisol interaction in depression and other neurological diseases: an alternative hypothesis. *Psychoneuroendocrinology.* 2007;32(7):854–855.

13. Lopez AD, Murray CC. The global burden of disease, 1990–2020. *Nat Med.* 1998;4(11):1241–1243.

14. Brown LC, Majumdar SR, Newman SC, et al. History of depression increases risk of type 2 diabetes in younger adults. *Diabetes Care.* 2005;28:1063–1067.

15. Carnethon MR, Kinder LS, Fair JM, et al. Symptoms of depression as a risk factor for incident diabetes: findings from the National Health and Nutrition Examination Epidemiologic Follow-up Study, 1971–1992. *Am J Epidemiol.* 2003;158:416–423.

16. Barnard KD, Skinner TC, Peveler R. The prevalence of co-morbid depression in adults with type 1 diabetes: systematic literature review. *Diabet Med.* 2006;23 (4):445.

17. Lloyd CE, Zgibor J, Wilson RR, et al. Cross-cultural comparisons of anxiety and depression in adults with type 1 diabetes. *Diabetes Metab Res Rev.* 2003; 19(5):401–407.

18. Anderson RJ, Freedland KE, Clouse RE, et al. The prevalence of comorbid depression in adults with diabetes: a meta-analysis. *Diabetes Care.* 2001;24(6): 1069–1078.

19. Ali S, Stone MA, Peters JL, et al. The prevalence of co-morbid depression in adults with type 2 diabetes: a systematic review and meta-analysis. *Diabet Med.* 2006;23(11):1165–1173.

20. Maraldi C, Volpato S, Penninx BW, et al. Diabetes mellitus, glycemic control, and incident depressive symptoms among 70- to 79-year-old persons: the health, aging, and body composition study. *Arch Intern Med.* 2007;167(11):1137–1144.

21. Hood KK, Huestis S, Maher A, et al. Depressive symptoms in children and adolescents with type 1 diabetes: association with diabetes-specific characteristics. *Diabetes Care.* 2006;29(6):1389–1391.

22. Knol MJ, Twisk JWR, Beekman ATF, et al. Depression as a risk factor for the onset of type 2 diabetes mellitus. A meta-analysis. *Diabetologia.* 2006;49(5):837–845.

23. Kooy FH. Hyperglycaemia in mental disorders. *Brain.* 1919;42(3):214–290.

24. Raphael T, Parsons JP. Blood sugar studies in dementia praecox and manic-depressive insanity. *Arch Neurol Psychiatry.* 1921;5:687–709.

25. Freeman H, Rodnick EH, Shakow D, et al. The carbohydrate tolerance of mentally disturbed soldiers. *Psychosom Med.* 1944;6(4):311–317.
26. Doroshow DB. Performing a cure for schizophrenia: insulin coma therapy on the wards. *J Hist Med Allied Sci.* 2007;62(2):213–243.
27. Kohen D. Diabetes mellitus and schizophrenia: historical perspective. *Br J Psychiatry.* 2004;184(47):s64–6.
28. Juvonen H, Reunanen A, Haukka J, et al. Incidence of schizophrenia in a nationwide cohort of patients with type 1 diabetes mellitus. *Arch Gen Psychiatry.* 2007;64(8):894–899.
29. Wild S, Roglic G, Green A, et al. Global prevalence of diabetes: estimates for the year 2000 and projections for 2030. *Diabetes Care.* 2004;27(5):1047–1053.
30. Rouillon F, Sorbara F. Schizophrenia and diabetes: epidemiological data. *Eur Psychiatry.* 2005;20 Suppl 4:S345.
31. Basu A, Meltzer HY. Differential trends in prevalence of diabetes and unrelated general medical illness for schizophrenia patients before and after the atypical antipsychotic era. *Schizophr Res.* 2006;86(1–3):99–109.
32. De Hert M, van Winkel R, Van Eyck D, et al. Prevalence of diabetes, metabolic syndrome and metabolic abnormalities in schizophrenia over the course of the illness: a cross-sectional study. *Clin Practice Epidemiol Ment Health.* 2006;2:14–23.
33. van Winkel R, De Hert M, Van Eyck D, et al. Screening for diabetes and other metabolic abnormalities in patients with schizophrenia and schizoaffective disorder: evaluation of incidence and screening methods. *J Clin Psychiatry.* 2006;67(10):1493–1500.
34. Hennekens CH, Hennekens AR, Hollar D, et al. Schizophrenia and increased risks of cardiovascular disease. *Am Heart J.* 2005;150(6):1115–1121.
35. Chafetz L, White MC, Collins-Bride G, et al. The poor general health of the severely mentally ill: impact of schizophrenic diagnosis. *Community Ment Health J.* 2005;41(2):169.
36. Raphael T, Parsons JP. Blood sugar studies in dementia praecox and manic-depressive insanity. *Arch Neurol Psychiatry.* 1921;5:681–709.
37. Bowman KM, Kasanin J. The sugar content of blood in emotional states. *Arch Neurol Psychiatry.* 1929;21:342–362.
38. Whitehorn JC. The blood sugar in relation to emotional reactions. *Am J Psychiatry.* 1934;90:987–1005.
39. Gildea EF, McLean VL, Man EB. Oral and Intravenous dextrose tolerance curves of patients with manic-depressive psychosis. *Arch Neurol Psychiatry.* 1943;49:852–859.
40. van der Velde CD, Gordon MW. Manic-depressive illness, diabetes mellitus and lithium carbonate. *Arch Gen Psychiatry.* 1969;21:478–485.
41. Lilliker S. Prevalence of diabetes in a manic-depressive population. *Compr Psychiatry.* 1980;21:270–275.
42. McIntyre RS, Konarski JZ, Misener VL, et al. Bipolar disorder and diabetes mellitus: epidemiology, etiology, and treatment implications. *Ann Clin Psychiatry.* 2005;17(2):83–93.
43. Kawamoto T, Horikawa Y, Tanaka T, et al. Genetic variations in the WFS1 gene in Japanese with type 2 diabetes and bipolar disorder. *Mol Genet Metab.* 2004 Jul;82(3):238–245.
44. Harrison PJ. The neuropathology of primary mood disorder. *Brain.* 2002 Jul;125(Pt 7):1428–1449.

45. Daban C, Vieta E, Mackin P, et al. Hypothalamic-pituitary-adrenal axis and bipolar disorder. *Psychiatr Clin North Am.* 2005 Jun;28(2):469–480.
46. Cassidy F, Ahearn E, Carroll BJ. Elevated frequency of diabetes mellitus in hospitalized manic-depressive patients. *Am J Psychiatry.* 1999;156:1417–1420.
47. Kilbourne AM, Cornelius JR, Han X, et al. Burden of general medical conditions among individuals with bipolar disorder. Bipolar Disord. 2004 Oct;6(5):368–373.
48. Regenold WT, Thapar RK, et al. Increased prevalence of type 2 diabetes mellitus among psychiatric inpatients with bipolar I affective and schizoaffective disorders independent of psychotropic drug use. *J Affect Disord.* 2002;70(1):19–26.
49. Ruzickova M, Slaney C, Garnham J, et al. Clinical features of bipolar disorder with and without comorbid diabetes mellitus. *Can J Psychiatry.* 2003;48:458–461.
50. McIntyre RS, Soczynska JK, Beyer JL, et al. Medical comorbidity in bipolar disorder: re-prioritizing unmet needs. *Curr Opin Psychiatry.* 2007 Jul;20(4):406–416.
51. Azziz R, Woods KS, Reyna R, et al. The prevalence and features of the polycystic ovary syndrome in an unselected population. *J Clin Endocrinol Metab.* 2004 Jun;89(6):2745–2749.
52. Guzick, DS. Cardiovascular risk in PCOS. *J Clin Endocrinol Metab.* 2004; Aug;89(8):3694–3695.
53. The Rotterdam ESHRE/ASRM-Sponsored PCOS Consensus Workshop Group. Consensus on diagnostic criteria and long-term health risks related to polycystic ovary syndrome (PCOS). *Hum Reprod.* 2003;19:41–47.
54. Solomon CG. The epidemiology of polycystic ovary syndrome. Prevalence and associated disease risks. *Endocrinol Metab Clin North Am.* 1999;28:247–263.
55. Ehrmann DA. Polycystic ovary syndrome. *N Engl J Med.* 2005;352:1223–1236.
56. Herzog AG. Menstrual disorders in women with epilepsy. Neurology. 2006;66 (6 suppl 3):S23–28.
57. O'Donovan C, Kusumakar V, Graves GR, et al. Menstrual abnormalities and polycystic ovary syndrome in women taking valproate for bipolar mood disorder. *J Clin Psychiatry.* 2002;63: 322–330.
58. Klipstein KG, Goldberg JF. Screening for bipolar disorder in women with polycystic ovary syndrome: a pilot study. *J Affect Disord.* 2006 Apr;91(2-3):205–209.
59. Rasgon NL, Altshuler LL, Fairbanks L, et al. Reproductive function and risk for PCOS in women treated for bipolar disorder. Bipolar Disord. 2005 Jun;7(3):246–259.
60. Ernst CL, Goldberg JF. The reproductive safety profile of mood stabilizers, atypical antipsychotics, and broad-spectrum psychotropics. *J Clin Psychiatry.* 2002; 63(suppl 4):42–55.
61. Rasgon NL, Altshuler LL, Gudeman D, et al. Medication status and the polycystic ovarian syndrome in women with bipolar disorder: a preliminary report. *J Clin Psychiatry.* 2000;61:173–178.
62. Freeman MP, Gelenberg AJ. Bipolar disorder in women: reproductive events and treatment considerations. Acta Psychiatr Scand. 2005 Aug;112(2):88–96.
63. Ehrmann DA, Barnes RB, Rosenfield RL, et al. Prevalence of impaired glucose tolerance and diabetes in women with polycystic ovary syndrome. *Diabetes Care.* 1999;22:141–146.
64. Legro RS, Kunselman AR, Dodson WC, et al. Prevalence and predictors of risk for type 2 diabetes mellitus and impaired glucose tolerance in polycystic ovary syndrome: a prospective, controlled study in 254 affected women. *J Clin Endocrinol Metab.* 1999;84:165–169.

CHAPTER 2

The Cost of Diabetes

Gale Z. Feldman

Overview

In 2003, the United States spent approximately $1.66 trillion on health care expenditures.[1] Spending for health care is outpacing the growth of the gross domestic product (GDP) and is expected to account for 17.7% of the GDP by 2012, up from 14.1% in 2001. Chronic health conditions, such as cardiovascular diseases and diabetes, account for more than 75% of national medical care costs.[2]

Diabetes alone represents 11% of U.S. health care expenditures.[3] With 14.6 million individuals living with diabetes in 2005 and an additional 6.2 million individuals who are undiagnosed, direct and indirect costs related to the treatment of diabetes are increasing.[4,5] During the past decade, diabetes ranked sixth among the 15 most expensive medical conditions treated in the United States and second in terms of median direct costs per person receiving treatment.[6] Annual costs significantly increased from $98 billion in 1997 to $132 billion in 2002;[3] adjusted for inflation, this was approximately $149 billion in 2005.[7] Given the current prevalence of diabetes in the United States, the total economic cost of diabetes could rise to $156 billion by 2010 and $192 billion (in 2002 dollars) by 2020.[3] Considering the projected increasing rates of obesity and diabetes partnered with escalating health care costs, the actual economic burden is likely to be significantly higher in future years.[4]

Of the $132 billion in expenditures attributed to diabetes in 2002, $91.8 billion was attributed to direct medical costs, more than doubling from $44 billion in 1997. Direct medical expenditures comprised $23.2 billion for diabetes care, $24.6 billion for chronic complications attributable to diabetes, and $44.1 billion for excess prevalence of general medical conditions. Per capita, medical expenditures total an average of $13,243 for individuals diagnosed with diabetes compared with $2,560 for individuals without diabetes.[3] Individuals with diabetes have medical expenditures approximately 2.4 times higher than individuals without diabetes (calculated using an age-adjusted per capita expenditure of $5,642 after controlling for differences in demographic characteristics).[3]

In addition, people with diabetes are at greater risk for temporary incapacity (defined as lost workdays and bed days), permanent disability, and premature mortality. The indirect costs of diabetes represent 30% of the total expenditures related to diabetes in 2002. The $39.8 billion in indirect costs includes $4.5 million for lost workdays, $6.3 million in restricted activity days, $7.5 million in permanent disability, and $21.6 for premature mortality.[3]

Indirect Costs

The economic loss in the United States due to diabetes was almost $40 billion in 2002 due to lost work time, disability, and premature mortality; this represents a considerable national economic burden. With a projected 17% increase in the total population and a 44% increase in individuals diagnosed with diabetes by 2020, the economic burden associated with indirect costs of diabetes may increase to $54 billion by 2020.[3] In addition to the impact on the national economy, employers face an economic burden due to decreased productivity secondary to diabetes. In 1997, diabetes accounted for an estimated 55 million disability days per year for individuals younger than age 65 years of age[8] and a one-third reduction in earning due to reduced work force participation, with an annual loss of $3,700 to $8,700 per person with diabetes.[9]

Lost Work Days/Bed Days: The economic impact to employers and the nation due to temporary incapacity can be measured by both lost workdays and the number of bed days. Lost workdays are defined as the number of days an individual is unable to participate in work or business because of diabetes-related morbidity. Bed days are defined as the number of days in which an individual is bedridden more than one-half day (including hospital stays) because of diabetes-related complications.

During the past decade, of the 15 most costly medical conditions, diabetes ranked eighth in terms of contributing to lost workdays and third in terms of contributing to bed days. In 1996, diabetes contributed to 210.5 million bed days and 27.5 million lost workdays.[10] On average, men with diabetes had 3.1 more lost workdays and 7.9 more bed days per year compared with men without diabetes. Similarly, women with diabetes had 0.6 more lost workdays and 8.1 more bed days than women without diabetes.[3] In 2002, the economic loss related to lost days of work and bed days totaled $10.8 billion (using an estimated $168 per day of earnings, the average for people with diabetes, in which a bed day equals 40% of the cost of a lost workday).[3] A 2002 study using claims from a nationwide Fortune 100 company with more than 100,000 beneficiaries, including industrial, service, and professional employees, demonstrated that mean annual work loss costs for employees with diabetes ranged from 1.7 to 2.2 times that of matched control employees. This accounted for losses ranging from an average of $1,095 to $1,448 per employee with diabetes compared with

$520 to $805 per employee without diabetes.[11] The sample used was representative of the U. S. population in terms of diabetes prevalence from 1996 to 1998.

Disability: Causes of disability for people with diabetes include amputations, loss of vision, renal failure, cardiovascular disease, and other physical problems that can limit earning potential or preclude individuals from gainful employment. During the past decade, diabetes was ranked second of the fifteen most costly medical conditions contributing to activities of daily living (ADL) and instrumental activities of daily living (IADL) impairment. ADL is a measurement of physical functioning, as related to activities such as eating, bathing, dressing, toileting, transferring, and continence. IADL, on the other hand, relates to more complex life activities such as light housework, laundry, meal preparation, transportation, grocery shopping, telephoning, medication management, and money management. In 1996, diabetes contributed to 1.95 million cases of ADL/IADL impairment.[10] Diabetes was accountable for 176,000 cases of disability at an annual cost of $7.5 billion. Using data from the Social Security Administration in 2002, an estimated 122,000 individuals 18–64 years of age received Social Security Disability Insurance (SSDI) benefits where diabetes was listed as the primary reason for disability. In addition, another 109,000 individuals received SSDI benefits where diabetes was listed as the secondary reason for disability, with cardiovascular disease, renal disease, and other diagnoses listed as the primary basis. Aggregating the data results in an estimated 176,475 person-years of permanent disability attributed to diabetes with an average of $42,462 in earnings lost per person per year.[3]

Disability claims are an economic burden for both employers and employees with diabetes. In 1997, diabetes accounted for 14 million lost disability days and an average of 8.3 days off from work per year compared with 1.7 days off from work for people without diabetes or other chronic conditions.[5] A 2002 nationwide workplace study of a Fortune 100 company demonstrated that the relative likelihood of an employee having a minimum of one disability claim was 33% for employees with diabetes versus 20% for employees without diabetes. The mean duration of a disability claim was 41 ± 98 days for employees with diabetes versus 22 ± 73 days for matched control employees. The study population was representative of the United States population in terms of diabetes prevalence from 1996 to 1998.[11] A 2004 cross-sectional and longitudinal study of data from the Health and Retirement Study demonstrated that the cumulative risk of incident disability over an 8-year period was 21.3% for individuals with diabetes versus 9.3% for those without diabetes. This study examined a cohort of adults ranging in age from 51 to 61 years from 1992 through 2000. In the same period, employees with diabetes reporting disability lost an average of $22,100 compared with employees without diabetes.[12]

Table 2.1 summarizes the morbidity costs attributed to diabetes.

Table **2.1** Morbidity costs attributable to diabetes, 2002			
Cause of permanent disability with diabetes listed as the primary or secondary basis of disability	Attributed disability cases	Percent of total attributed cases	Value of lost productivity (billions of dollars)
Diabetes	121,893	69	5.2
Cardiovascular disease	12,110	7	0.5
Renal disease	3,887	2	0.2
Other diagnoses	38,584	22	1.6
Total	176,475	100	7.5

From Hogan P, Dall T, Nikolov P. Economic costs of diabetes in the United States in 2002. *Diabetes Care*. 2003;26:917–932, with permission.

Mortality: Diabetes is the sixth leading cause of death in the United States.[5] Nationally, the age-adjusted death rate for diabetes is 75 deaths per 100,000 population, with 8.8 deaths per 1,000 population related to diabetes (listed as either a primary or subsequent cause of death).[13] In 2002, diabetes contributed to an estimated 186,000 premature deaths, according to the Centers for Disease Control and Prevention: Multiple Cause of Death for ICD-9 data. Overall, the risk of death among people with diabetes is about twice that of people without diabetes.[14]

Premature death resulted in 2.5 million years of life lost prematurely from diabetes.[3] Mortality-related productivity costs are the estimated value of lost future earnings and incorporate both the number and timing of premature deaths attributable to diabetes. The value of lost productivity from premature mortality is $21.6 billion dollars,[3] representing 54% of indirect costs and 16% of the total direct and indirect costs related to diabetes.[14]

Comorbidities related to diabetes are often the primary cause of mortality. Cardiovascular disease accounts for 58% of all deaths related to diabetes, with 108,000 deaths per year and $10.3 billion in lost productivity.[3] Adults with diabetes suffer death rates due to cardiovascular complications two to four times higher than do adults without diabetes.[5] Cerebrovascular disease accounts for 2% of deaths related to diabetes, with 4,000 deaths per year and $305 million in lost productivity. An estimated 2,000 deaths related to renal disease are attributed to diabetes, with $273 million in lost productivity.[3] Age-adjusted mortality rates for people with renal disease related to diabetes are more than 2.5 times the rates for individuals without diabetes.[15]

Refer to Table 2.2 for a summary of mortality costs attributed to diabetes.

Table **2.2**	Mortality costs attributable to diabetes, 2002			
Primary cause of death	Deaths attributed to diabetes (thousands)	Percent of total U.S. deaths	Total lost years (thousands)	Value of lost productivity (millions of dollars)
Diabetes	72	100	1,080	10,622
Renal disease	2	6	31	273
Cerebrovascular disease	4	12	54	305
Cardiovascular disease	108	19	1,357	10,358
Grand total	186	NA	2,522	21,558

From Hogan P, Dall T, Nikolov P. Economic costs of diabetes in the United States in 2002. *Diabetes Care.* 2003;26:917–932, with permission.

Direct Costs

The overall population living with diabetes carries a disproportionate share of health care expenditures. Of the 15 most costly medical conditions in the United States, diabetes ranks ranked sixth in total direct medical expenditures, despite the fact that it ranks eleventh in total number of individuals diagnosed with a medical condition.[6] Although people with diabetes comprise just slightly more than 4% of the U.S. population,[3] 19% of every dollar spent on health care (including hospitalizations, outpatient and physician visits, ambulance services, nursing home care, home health care, hospice, and medication/glucose control agents) is incurred by individuals with diabetes; 11% of health care costs are spent on conditions specifically related to diabetes.[3] More than $91.8 billion in direct medical expenditures is attributable to the treatment of diabetes and related complications. Approximately $160 billion in direct health care costs is incurred by people with diabetes for all medical conditions (including conditions unrelated to diabetes), representing nearly one-fifth of the total U.S. expenditures for hospital institutional care (including hospital inpatient days), outpatient care, ambulance services, diabetic medications, home health care, and hospice. Expenditures attributable directly to diabetes and its complications include $40.3 billion for hospital inpatient care, representing 9% of the U.S. total, $13.9 for nursing home care, and $10 billion for physician office visits. The cost of oral agents to lower glucose, insulin, and insulin-related supplies totals almost $12 billion.[3]

For certain services, diabetes accounts for a disproportionate share of expenses. In 2002, diabetes-related hospitalizations totaled 16.9 million days and accounted for 62.6 million physician office visits, 5.9 million hospital outpatient visits, and 4.8 million emergency department visits. Diabetes is responsible for 18% of total U.S. expenditures for home health care (44.2 million visits per year), 15% for nursing home care (82.3 million visits), and 14% for hospice care (more than 5 million hospice care days).[3] Overall, the annual per capita health care expenditures are 2.4 times greater for individuals diagnosed with diabetes than for those without diabetes.[3]

Comorbidities

Complications associated with diabetes can lead to significant costs to individuals and the health care system. People with diabetes are at greater risk for cardiovascular disease, renal disease, neurological disorders, peripheral vascular disease, endocrine/metabolic complications, and ophthalmological problems. In 1997, only 8% of the population with a medical claim of diabetes was treated for diabetes alone. Other conditions influenced health care spending, with 13.8% of the population with one other condition, 11.2% with two comorbidities, and 67% with three or more related conditions.[6]

Patients with diabetes who suffer from comorbid conditions related to diabetes have a greater impact on health services compared with those patients who do not have comorbid conditions. Treatment for comorbid conditions related to diabetes accounts for 95% of inpatient hospitalizations for diabetes, 84% of physician office visits, 93% of emergency department visits, and 77% of hospital outpatient visits. In addition, conditions associated with diabetes are responsible for 69% of nursing home days, 62% of home health visits, and 98% of hospice care of total nursing home care days for the population with diabetes.[3]

Significant proportions of costs associated with diabetes are directly related to complications and comorbid conditions. Overall, comorbid conditions and complications are responsible for 75% of total medical expenditures for diabetes. Costs of more than $68.6 billion are attributed to the treatment of comorbid conditions and complications, with general medical conditions contributing the greatest expense across all service categories. Cardiovascular disease is the most costly complication of diabetes, accounting for $17.6 billion in health care and more than 19% of total expenditures directed toward diabetes (Table 2.3).[3]

Cardiovascular Disease: Heart disease and stroke are the largest contributors to mortality for individuals with diabetes; these two conditions are responsible for 65% of deaths. Death rates from heart disease in adults with diabetes are two to four times higher than in adults without diabetes. Likewise, in adults with diabetes, the risk of stroke is two to four times higher, and the risk of death from stroke is 2.8 times higher. Among women with diabetes, there has been a 23% increase in the death rate from heart disease over the past 30 years compared with a 27% decrease among women without diabetes. Among men with diabetes, there has been only a 13% decrease in deaths due to heart disease compared with a 36% decrease in men without diabetes.[5]

The prevalence of cardiovascular disease is almost 75% greater in adults with diabetes compared to adults without diabetes, with a risk ratio of 1.74.

Table **2.3**   Health care expenditures attributable to diabetes, by medical condition and type of service, 2002[a] (in millions of dollars)

Medical condition	Inpatient days	Office visits	Outpatient visits	Emergency visits	Nursing home days	Home health visits	Hospice care days	Other[b]	Total
Diabetes	2,043	1,591	761	140	4,263	1,504	13	12,916	23,231
Neurological symptoms	1,096	104	26	29	1,339	96	4	52	2,748
Peripheral vascular disease	746	54	27	14	159	89	1	31	1,121
Cardiovascular disease	9,740	2,093	767	312	2,128	620	74	1,892	17,626
Renal complications	977	157	62	75	438	71	6	92	1,879
Endocrine/metabolic complications	38	188	52	2	18	3	0	126	426
Ophthalmological complications	11	241	61	9	2	7	0	92	422
Other complications	212	28	9	19	27	9	0	14	318
General medical conditions	25,473	5,578	1,549	1,562	5,504	1,531	445	2,447	44,091
Total	40,337	10,033	3,315	2,162	13,878	3,930	543	17,662	91,861

[a]In millions of dollars.
[b]Includes ambulance services, outpatient medications, oral agents, insulin, and supplies.
From Hogan P, Dall T, Nikolov P. Economic costs of diabetes in the United States in 2002. *Diabetes Care*. 2003;26:917–932, with permission.

Table 2.4 Use, share, proportion, and expenditures attributable to diabetes for cardiovascular disease

Service	U.S. health care use (in thousands)	Share of total U.S. health care use[a]	Proportion of total U.S. health care use[b]	Health care expenditures by type of service (in millions of dollars)
Inpatient days	4,084	24	19	9,740
Nursing home days	12,628	15	19	2,128
Physician office visits	13,064	21	20	2,093
Emergency visits	690	14	20	312
Hospital outpatient visits	1,367	23	22	767
Home health visits	6,973	16	19	620
Hospice care days	698	14	19	74
Other[c]				1,892
Total				17,626

[a]Data are percentages. For example, of total inpatient days for diabetes, 24% were attributable to cardiovascular disease.
[b]Data are percentages. For example, 19% of all inpatient days for cardiovascular disease (as the primary condition) were attributable to diabetes.
[c]Includes ambulance services, outpatient medications, oral agents, insulin, and supplies.
Data from Hogan P, Dall T, Nikolov P. Economic costs of diabetes in the United States in 2002. *Diabetes Care.* 2003;26:917–932.

(95% confidence interval [CI] 1.68–1.82). Adults with diabetes are more than twice as likely to have multiple diagnoses related to macrovascular disease compared to patients without diabetes (risk ratio 2.12, 95% CI 1.97–2.26).[16] Although the prevalence of cardiovascular disease increases with age for both diabetics and nondiabetics, adults with diabetes have a significantly higher rate of disease. In adults younger than 45 years of age with diabetes, 5.2% were diagnosed with a cardiovascular condition compared with 1.3% of age-matched adults without diabetes. For adults older than 85 years of age, 61.4% of adults with diabetes had cardiovascular disease compared with 48.9% of age-matched adults without diabetes.[16]

Cardiovascular disease is the most costly complication of diabetes, accounting for $17.6 billion of annual direct medical costs for diabetes in 2002. Diabetes accounts for 19% to 22% of costs related to all incidences of cardiovascular disease. Similarly, cardiovascular disease accounts for more than 19% of total costs for diabetes.[3] Refer to Table 2.4 for a summary of expenditures attributable to diabetes for cardiovascular disease.

The management of macrovascular disease, such as heart attacks and strokes, represents the largest factor driving medical service use and related costs, accounting for 52% of costs to treat diabetes over a lifetime. The average costs of treating macrovascular disease are $24,330 of a total of $47,240 per person (in year 2000 dollars) over the course of a lifetime.[17] Moreover, macrovascular disease is an important determinant of cost at an earlier time than other complications, accounting for 85% of the cumulative costs during the first 5 years following diagnosis and 77% over the initial decade.[17]

The impact of cardiovascular disease is more severe on health and costs when cooccurring with diabetes. Individuals with cardiovascular disease and diabetes are much more likely to experience myocardial infarction and congestive heart failure compared with adults with a single diagnosis of cardiovascular disease, who are more susceptible to arrhythmias and other nonischemic cardiovascular conditions. Adults with diabetes are 2.78 times more likely to have a myocardial infarction and 2.71 times more likely to be diagnosed with congestive heart failure.[16] For individuals surviving one year following a myocardial infarction, the direct medical costs the year following the incident were $24,500 ($15,000–$50,000). For individuals surviving a stroke, the total costs for the year following the acute incident were $26,600 ($15,400–$44,900).[18]

Cardiovascular disease in the presence of diabetes affects not only cost but also the allocation of health care resources. Average annual individual costs attributed to the treatment of diabetes with cardiovascular disease were $10,172. Almost 51% of costs were for inpatient hospitalizations, 28% were for outpatient care, and 21% were for pharmaceuticals and related supplies. In comparison, the average annual costs for adults with diabetes and without cardiovascular disease were $4,402 for management and treatment of diabetes. Only 31.2% of costs were for inpatient hospitalizations, 40.3% were for outpatient care, and 28.6% were for pharmaceuticals.[16]

Reducing adverse health outcomes associated with cardiovascular disease in the presence of diabetes would significantly reduce costs, decrease mortality rates, and improve quality of life. Preventing and controlling hypertension reduces the risk of heart disease and stroke among people with diabetes by 33% to 50%. In general, for every 10–mm Hg reduction in systolic blood pressure, the risk of any complication related to diabetes is reduced by 12%. Management of cholesterolemia can reduce cardiovascular complications by 20% to 50%.[5] Better access to preventive care, earlier diagnoses, and intensive chronic disease management could potentially moderate national expenditures for health care services by reducing the largest driver of costs associated with complications of diabetes.

Peripheral Neuropathy and Amputation: Peripheral neuropathy and peripheral vascular disease are particularly debilitating complications related to diabetes, predisposing the feet to ulceration and lower extremity amputation. Some degree of diabetic peripheral neuropathy occurs in 12% to 50% of individuals with diabetes.[19] Of individuals with diabetes, 2% to 3% develop a foot ulcer during any given year. The lifetime incidence rate of lower extremity ulcers is 15% in the diabetic population.[20]

Deep foot ulcerations may be accompanied by cellulitis or osteomyelitis, increasing the risk of amputation of the toe, foot, or leg if ulcerations do not heal. The rate of amputation in individuals with diabetes is ten times higher than in those without diabetes.[5] Diabetic lower-extremity ulcers are responsible for 92,000 amputations each year,[21] accounting for more than 60% of all nontraumatic amputations.[5] The 10-year cumulative incidence of lower-extremity amputation is 7% in adults older than 30 years of age who are diagnosed with diabetes.[22] Within 5 years of the initial amputation, 28% to 51% of diabetic patients require a second leg amputation.[20] Following amputation, the 5-year survival rate is 27%.[23]

Diabetic peripheral neuropathy accounted for $10.1 billion of annual direct medical costs for type 2 diabetes in 2001.[19] Although neuropathy accounts for 9%[19] to 17%[17] of total national costs spent on diabetes, the individual cumulative cost over a lifetime is higher than for other conditions, with an average of more than $45,000 spent over a period of 30 years.[17] Per episode, costs for lower-limb ulcer-related health care are $13,179 ± $34,590.[24]

As many as 49% of individuals with diabetes have symptoms of diabetic peripheral neuropathy, with 6.2% of these individuals developing a lower extremity ulcer. The majority of annual costs associated with treating diabetic peripheral neuropathy are associated with treatment of ulcers; this accounts for $8.4 billion in health care expenditures. The total cost associated with lower-extremity amputation is $1.5 billion per year. Although the aggregated cost of lower-limb amputation is lower than the treatment of ulcerations, the burden of cost is greater; only 0.6% of individuals with neuropathic foot ulcers have lower-extremity amputations, whereas the $1.5 billion of the total cost of treatment (Table 2.5).[19]

Table 2.5	Prevalence and cost of diabetic peripheral neuropathy (DPN) and related complications			
Health state	Number of individuals with DPN and related complications	Prevalence of DPN and related complications	Mean weekly cost of DPN and related complications	Annual cost of DPN and related complications[a]
DPN	5,027,995	49%	$6	216
Neuropathic foot ulcer		6.8%		
Not infected	612,290	87.4% (of the 6.8% with an ulcer)	$179	5,698
With cellulitis	63,144	9.0% (of the 6.8% with an ulcer)	$473	1,552
With osteomyelitis	25,323	3.6%	$877	1,154
Amputation		0.6% (of the 6.8% with an ulcer)		
Toe	15,617	39% (of the 0.6% with an amputation)	$22,703	355
Foot	4,805	12% (of the 0.6% with an amputation)	$42,673	205
Leg	18,820	47% (of the 0.6% with an amputation)	$51,281	965

[a]Values in millions of dollars.

Data from Gordon A, Scuffham P, Shearer A, et al. The health care costs of diabetic peripheral neuropathy in the U.S. *Diabetes Care*. 2003;26:1790–1795.

Total ulcer-related costs averaged $13,179 per episode and increased with outcome severity. Ulcer-related costs per episode increased from $1,892 for superficial ulcers to $27,721 for treatment of gangrene and amputation. Across all levels, inpatient acute hospitalization represented the majority of the costs, averaging $10,188 per episode.[24]

Approximately 60% to 70% of diabetic foot ulcers are related to neuropathies and the remainder is a consequence of vascular disease leading to ischemia.[19] Ischemia and compromised circulation from peripheral vascular conditions can prolong ulcer healing and increase the risk of amputation.[25] As the severity of ulceration increases, so does the presence of inadequate vascular status, as well as the average cost of treatment and management of lower-extremity ulcers. The mean cost of treating ulcer-related complications for individuals with adequate vascular status was $5,218 across all levels of severity compared with $23,372 for adults with inadequate vascular status. Patients suffering from gangrene and/or lower-extremity amputation with inadequate vascular status incurred significantly higher costs, averaging $34,845 per episode. On average, costs were $18,154 higher for patients with inadequate vascular status compared with patients with adequate vascular status.[24]

Overall, inpatient hospitalization is a major driver of cost, accounting for 77% of expenditures associated with individual episodes of lower-extremity ulcers.[24] Episode costs increased with severity and were impacted by vascular status. The data accentuate the significance of early diagnosis and aggressive treatment to prevent hospitalization and ulcer progression.

End-Stage Renal Failure: The incidence and prevalence of end-stage renal failure (ESRD) have steadily increased over the past two decades. Between 1980 and 2001, the incidence increased by a factor of four, from 82 to 334 cases per million of the total U.S. population. The prevalence increased by a factor of five, from 271 to 1,400 per million.[26] Much of the increase in prevalence and incidence can be attributed to diabetes. Diabetic nephropathy is the national leading cause of ESRD.

Between 1982 and 1992, the prevalence of diabetes as the underlying cause of ESRD increased from 27% to 36%.[26] By 2003, diabetes accounted for 37% of individuals being treated for renal disease in the United States. Of 452,957 adults undergoing treatment for ESRD, 165,113 cases were attributed to diabetes. Diabetes is the leading cause of kidney failure, accounting for 44% of all newly diagnosed cases. In 2003, among 102,567 individuals newly diagnosed with ESRD, 45,330 of those with diabetes began treatment with chronic dialysis or a underwent kidney transplantation for ESRD.[26]

In a study examining the differences of costs between pre-onset of ESRD and postdiagnosis, results demonstrated that the monthly costs of treating nephropathy and related conditions ranged from $1,535 to $4,357 among patients with diabetes compared with $1,038 to $2,447 for patients without diabetes. However, in the month preceding diagnosis of ESRD, total monthly costs for all conditions more than doubled for individuals with diabetes to $9,152 and more than tripled to $8,211 for individuals without diabetes. Costs escalated sharply following the onset of ESRD, with costs being similar in both groups ($26,507 and $26,789). Among the individuals with diabetes, costs specifically related to renal treatment increased from an average of $590 in the month preceding onset of ESRD to $20,436 immediately after the diagnosis.[27]

Total adjusted per-patient costs increased by 150% from $38,041 to $96,014 for individuals with diabetes and ESRD over a 24-month period (12 months before and after the diagnosis). Adjusted total annual costs specifically for renal-related services more than quintupled from $15,442 prior to diagnosis to $80,414 after diagnosis. Adjusted total annual costs were significantly higher for patients with diabetes compared with those without diabetes. In the period preceding diagnosis, total annual costs were 69% higher for patients with diabetes ($38,041) compared to patients without diabetes ($22,538). After the diagnosis of ESRD, costs were 79% higher for patients with diabetes ($96,014) compared to patients without diabetes ($53,653).

Health care expenditures for renal complications contribute 2% of the total direct medical costs for treating diabetes. The total direct medical cost for renal complications totals almost $1.9 billion per year. The majority of the cost is attributed to inpatient hospitalization, accounting for 52% of total expenditures for treatment of renal complications. Other expenses include $438 million spent on nursing home care and $157 million for physician office visits.[3]

The amount of direct medical costs for ESRD attributed to diabetes is substantial. The total adjusted costs in a 24-month period were 76% higher among ESRD patients with diabetes compared with those without diabetes. The adjusted change in costs from pre- to post-onset of ERSD was almost twice as high among patients with diabetes, with a change in mean costs of $57,973 for those with diabetes compared with $31,115 for those without diabetes. Nearly one half of the costs of ESRD are due to diabetes.[27]

These data emphasize the importance of preventing or delaying the onset and progression of ESRD. Through early detection, the impact of nephropathy can be decreased by managing hypertension and maintaining glycemic control. Each percentage drop in glycosylated hemoglobin, or A_{1c}, reduces the risk of microvascular complications, including kidney disease, by 40%. Furthermore, reduction in blood pressure can reduce the decline in kidney function by 30% to 70%.[5]

Table 2.6 summarizes the use, share, proportion and expenditures attributable to renal complications of diabetes.

Obesity: More than 133 million adults in the United States are considered overweight or obese based on their body mass index (BMI).[28] Of all adults, 68.5 million are considered to be overweight (BMI = $25-29.9$ Kg/m^2) and 64.7 million are considered to be obese (BMI ≥30 kg/m^2). The prevalence of overweight and obese adults has steadily increased from 44.8% of the total

Table **2.6**	Use, share, proportion, and expenditures attributable to renal complications of diabetes			
Service	U.S. health care use (in thousands)	Share of total U.S. health care use	Proportion of total U.S. health care use	Health care expenditures by type of service (in millions of dollars)
Inpatient days	410	2	10	977
Nursing home days	2,600	3	20	438
Physician office visits	980	2	8	157
Emergency visits	166	3	7	75
Hospital outpatient visits	11	2	8	62
Home health visits	803	2	12	71
Hospice care days	52	1	10	6
Other[a]				92
Total				**1,879**

[a]Includes ambulance services, outpatient medications, oral agents, insulin, and supplies.
Data from Hogan P, Dall T, Nikolov P. Economic costs of diabetes in the United States in 2002. *Diabetes Care.* 2003;26:917–932.

population in 1960 to 66.3% of the total population in 2002, and the prevalence of obesity has more than doubled, increasing from 13.3% to 32.2%.[29] Morbid obesity (BMI $\geq$40 kg/m^2) has increased from 0.8% in 1960 to 4.9% in 2002.[30]

Obesity is associated with increased mortality rates, with a 10% to 50% increased risk of death from all causes in obese individuals compared with healthy-weight individuals (BMI = 18–24.9 kg/m^2). The majority of increased risk is related to cardiovascular disease.[31] Relative to healthy-weight individuals, obesity is associated with approximately 112,000 excess deaths per year in the United States.[32] Estimates of the number of years of life lost related to weight status range as high as 20 years for specific age and racial/ethnic groups, with a 10% to 40% reduction in total life expectancy.[33]

Obesity is associated with many chronic diseases, including type 2 diabetes, cardiovascular disease, several types of cancer (endometrial, postmenopausal breast, kidney, and colon), musculoskeletal disorders, sleep apnea, arthritis, and gallbladder disease.[34] As weight increases, the prevalence and risk of disease also increases. In normal-weight men and women, the prevalence of diabetes in the population is 2.03% and 2.38% respectively; however, diabetes affects 10.65% of men and 19.89% of women with a BMI greater than 40 kg/m^2.[34] Compared with adults of normal weight, those with a BMI of 40 kg/m^2 or higher had an odds ratio of 7.37 (95% CI, 6.39–8.50) for diabetes, 6.38 (95% CI, 5.67–7.17) for hypertension, 1.88 (95% CI, 1.67–2.13) for cholesterolemia, and 4.41 (95% CI, 3.91–4.97) and 4.19 (95% CI, 3.68–4.76) for fair or poor health.[35]

As disease and risk conditions increase with excess weight and obesity, so does the utilization of health care resources and health care expenditures. Overall, 9.1% of total health care expenditures in the United States may be attributed to excessive body weight and obesity.[36] The total direct health care costs for all conditions of adults with a BMI >30 kg/m^2 was determined to be $238.3 billion. Of the total cost, $102.2 billion is attributed to 15 comorbid conditions incurred by obese adults (Table 2.7).[37] The public sector, through Medicare and Medicaid, may be responsible for up to 50% of the costs associated with comorbidities and obesity.[36] Obesity may account for up to a 36% increase in costs for inpatient and ambulatory care, which is greater than smoking, aging 20 years, or excessive alcohol consumption.[38]

Overall, the amount spent on treatment of disease related to obesity represented 27% to 31% of total direct costs of specific conditions. The impact of obesity on expenditures most greatly affected costs associated with cardiovascular disease and diabetes. Obesity was responsible for 30% of the costs attributed to cardiovascular disease for a total of $30.6 billion and for 43% of the costs of diabetes for a total of $20.5 billion.[37] In addition to greater costs associated with increased utilization of physician services and inpatient hospitalization, obese individuals have high annual costs for medications, particularly for the treatment of diabetes and cardiovascular disease. Obese individuals may pay almost 77% more for medications compared with nonobese individuals.[39]

Obesity significantly affects indirect costs, with businesses and employers bearing a sizeable portion of costs associated with obesity, including lost productivity and increased costs of health and disability insurance. In 1994, the estimated cost of obesity to U.S. businesses was $12.7 billion, including $2.6 billion related to mild obesity and $10.1 billion attributed to moderate to severe obesity. Expenditures associated with health insurance accounted for $7.7 billion of the total, representing 43% of all spending by U.S. businesses on coronary heart disease, hypertension, type 2 diabetes, hypercholesterolemia, stroke, gallbladder disease, osteoarthritis of the knee, and endometrial cancer. In addition, businesses spent $2.4 billion on paid sick leave, $1.8 billion on life insurance, and $800 million on disability insurance.[40]

Obese employees were more than 1.74 times more likely to experience high-level absenteeism, defined as seven or more absences in the previous 6 months, and 1.61 times more likely to experience moderate absenteeism than

Table **2.7**	Obesity costs in relation to comorbidities (1999 dollars in billions)		
Disease	Direct cost of obesity	Direct cost of disease	Direct cost of obesity as percentage of total direct cost of disease
Arthritis	$7.4	$23.1	32%
Breast cancer	$2.1	$10.2	21%
Heart disease	$30.6	$101.8	30%
Colorectal cancer	$2.0	$10.0	20%
Diabetes (type 2)	$20.5	$47.2	43%
Endometrial cancer	$0.6	$2.5	24%
ESRD	$3.0	$14.9	20%
Gallstones	$3.5	$7.7	45%
Hypertension	$9.6	$24.5	39%
Liver disease	$3.4	$9.7	35%
Low back pain	$3.5	$19.2	18%
Renal cell cancer	$0.5	$1.6	31%
Obstructive sleep apnea	$0.2	$0.4	50%
Stroke	$8.1	$29.5	27%
Urinary incontinence	$7.6	$29.2	26%
Total direct cost	**$102.2**	**$331.4**	**31%**

ESRD, end-stage renal disease.
From The Lewin Group–American Obesity Association. Costs of Obesity. 2002. http://www.obesity.org/treatment/cost.shtml. Copyright, The Obesity Society, with permission.

employees with normal weight.[41] According to National Health Interview Survey (NHIS) data from 1988 to 1994, the cost of lost productivity related to obesity increased 50% for a total of $3.9 billion in 1994, representing 39.2 million days of lost work. Contributing to lost productivity were 239 million restricted activity days and 89.5 million bed days, amounting to a substantial increase of 36% and 28%, respectively, compared to six years prior. The number of physician visits attributed to obesity increased 88% to 67.6 million physician visits during the same time period.[42] Excess weight is a risk factor for a large number of diseases and chronic conditions, significantly affecting the health, quality of life, and life expectancy of the U.S. population.

Depression: Individuals suffering from chronic disease, such as diabetes or cardiovascular disease, have an increased risk of depression compared to the overall population. In 2004, 42.5% of adults with diabetes reported at least one day of poor mental health in the previous month, and 32.1% reported poor mental and physical health. The odds of major depression in adults with diabetes are approximately twice as great as in those without diabetes.[43] Eleven to fifteen percent of all patients with type 2 diabetes meet the criteria established in the *Diagnostic and Statistical Manual of Mental Disorders*, 4th edition (DSM IV) for major depression.[43] As many as two-thirds of patients with diabetes and major depression have been ill with depression for more than 2 years.[44]

Among patients with diabetes, minor and major depression are associated with increased mortality. For individuals with diabetes, minor depression is associated with a 1.67-fold increase in mortality, and major depression is associated with a 2.3-fold increase in mortality. During a 3-year period, approximately 13.6% of deaths were attributed to patients with diabetes who suffered from minor depression and 11.9% of deaths to patients with major depression, compared with 8.3% of patients with diabetes but without depression.[45]

Depression may be associated with increased mortality due to biological and behavioral factors. Depression has been linked to decreased adherence to self-care regimens (exercise, diet, and cessation of smoking) in patients with diabetes, as well as to the use of diabetes control medications such as oral hypoglycemic, lipid-lowering, and antihypertensive prescriptions.[46] Patients with diabetes and depression are twice as likely to have three or more cardiac risk factors such as smoking, obesity, sedentary lifestyle, or A_{1c} >8.0% compared with patients with diabetes alone.[47]

Patients with depression are significantly more likely to have macrovascular and microvascular complications. Depression may increase the risk of complications associated with diabetes due to lack of adherence with self-care recommendations, as well as possibly due to neuroendocrine[48] and autonomic nervous system complications[49] associated with depression. Depression may be associated with mortality due to poor glucose regulation based on hypothalamic-pituitary axis abnormalities.[50] Furthermore, in patients with depression there is an increased risk of myocardial infarction[51] due to increased platelet adhesiveness and aggregation, increased markers of inflammatory response such as C-reactive protein levels, endothelial dysfunction, and increased sympathoadrenal activity.[49]

Depression is a major contributor to costs resulting in potentially serious complications for individuals with chronic disease including diabetes. In 2000, $83.1 billion was attributed to depression-related conditions (without presence of comorbid conditions). Of the cost related to the treatment of depression, $26.1 billion (31%) was attributed to direct medical costs, $5.4 billion (7%) were mortality costs related to suicide, and $51.5 billion (62%) were related to lost productivity in the workplace. While the treatment rate for depression increased more than 50% from 1990 to 2000, the economic burden remained relatively stable, rising by only 7% despite a dramatic increase in the proportion of individuals with depression receiving treatment.[52]

The costs for individuals with both major depression and diabetes are 4.5 times greater than for those with diabetes alone.[53] Individuals with diabetes

Table **2.8**	Mean and median annual non–mental health-related Medicare payments for diabetes and depression		
	Claimants with diabetes (no major depression)	Claimants with major depression (no diabetes)	Claimants with diabetes and major depression
Unadjusted mean (updated to 2001 dollars)	$10,358	$13,153	$25,360
Median	$2,453	$3,956	$11,445

Data from Finkelstein EA, Bray JW, Chen H, et al. Prevalence and costs of major depression among elderly claimants with diabetes. *Diabetes Care.* 2003;26:415–420.

presenting with greater depressive symptoms are confronted with 51% to 86% higher costs.[54] Medicare claimants with diabetes and major depression have 21% greater annual non–mental health-related payments and 23% greater payment for nonmental health physician services. On average, in 1997, these claimants with diabetes and major depression had an average of 14 additional non–mental health-related physician services.[55] In addition, these claimants are no more likely to be admitted to the hospital than claimants with diabetes who do not carry the diagnosis of major depression. However, of those admitted, claimants with diabetes and depression have an average of 17% more non–mental health-related inpatient days and 7% greater costs during their inpatient stay (Table 2.8).[55]

Costs related to lost productive work time from U.S. workers with depression are significant. On average, employees with depression reported an average decrease of 5.6 hours per week of productive work compared with 1.5 hours per week for employees without depression. Eighty-one percent of costs related to lost productive time were related to decreased performance. U.S. workers with depression cost employers an estimated $44 billion dollars per year in lost production time compared with peers without depression who attribute to an average of $13 billion per year, not including the labor costs associated with short and long tem disability.[56]

Schizophrenia: Individuals with schizophrenia often experience comorbid conditions, which become major drivers of health care costs related to the treatment of mental illness. The prevalence of obesity and diabetes is 1.5 to 2 times greater in patients with schizophrenia than in the general population.[57] Of adults with schizophrenia, 16% had diabetes and an additional 30.9% had impaired glucose tolerance.[58] Metabolic syndrome was present in 65% of individuals with schizophrenia,[59] which is three times greater than its occurrence in the general population.[60] The risk of cardiovascular ailments in patients with schizophrenia is also increased. Compared with the general population, patients with schizophrenia have a 1.5 times increased risk of arrhythmia, a 4 times increased risk of syncope, a 1.7 times increased risk of heart failure, a 2.1 times increased risk of stroke, and a 2.6 times increased risk of transient cerebral ischemia. In addition, they have a higher mortality rate from cardiovascular disease.[61]

Costs related to schizophrenia alone and with comorbidities have a significant impact on total health care costs. During 2001 and 2002, an estimated 571,000 adults with schizophrenia were residing in the community. During this period, direct medical expense accounted for $2.13 billion, including costs related to hospitalizations, physician visits, outpatient procedures, transportation for medical care, and prescriptions. Mean expense per patient was $3,726, with median expenses representing $1,748 per person.[62] The majority of expenses were associated with outpatient care, including 486,000 ambulatory and emergency department visits, accounting for 36.6% of the overall mean per-person costs for an annual total of $780 million.[62] The majority of adults with schizophrenia (503,000) utilized prescriptions related to their condition, accounting for $820 million of annual costs and 38.7% of per-person expenditures.[62] In 2001–2002, there were 51,000 home health care visits for individuals with schizophrenia, representing 11.8% of overall mean per-person expenditures and $250 million in annual costs. Inpatient care accounted for 13% of total health care expenditures for patients with schizophrenia, representing 47,000 adults who required hospitalization. Of overall mean per-person health care expenses, 13% was for hospitalization expenses, representing an average inpatient expense of $5856 for an annual total of $280 million per year (Table 2.9).[62]

Approximately two-thirds of people with schizophrenia also suffer from hypertension, cardiovascular disease, dyslipidemia, or diabetes. Approximately 83,000 people with schizophrenia and diabetes sought treatment in 2001 and 2002, for an average of $11,611 per person for all health care, compared with an average of $5,990 for treatment of schizophrenia with no comorbidity. Annual spending for the 165,000 adults with schizophrenia and hypertension totaled $12,292, which is more than twice that of spending for health care related to schizophrenia without comorbidities. Almost 23% of all adults with schizophrenia are also diagnosed with cardiovascular disease, totaling $10,415 per person for all health care expenses. About 79,000 people with schizophrenia were treated for dyslipidemia, for an average of $10,803 per person (Table 2.10).[62]

Common comorbidities significantly increase the costs of patients with schizophrenia. Associated comorbidities increase cost by 20% to 90% per year. When total health care spending is considered, the cost of treating schizophrenia with comorbidities is more than four times the cost of treating schizophrenia alone.[62]

Table 2.9 Annual direct health care spending for schizophrenia and related psychoses and percent distribution of spending by service site in community dwelling adults, 2001–2002

Site of service	Number of patients with an expense	Total ($ billions)	Median annual spending ($)	Mean ($)	Percent of overall mean	Stand error of mean ($)
Overall	571,000	2.13	1748	3726	100.0	562
Inpatient	47,000	0.28	0	483	13.0	185
Ambulatory/ emergency care	486,000	0.78	346	1363	36.6	280
Prescription drugs	503,000	0.82	409	1442	38.7	296
Home health care	51	0.25	0	439	11.8	245

From McDonald M, Hertz RP, Lustik MB, et al. Healthcare spending among community-dwelling adults with schizophrenia. *Am J of Manag Care.* 2005;11(suppl):S242–S247, with permission.

Table 2.10 Annual spending per person with schizophrenia or related psychoses, by comorbidity category in community-dwelling adults, 2001–2002

Comorbidity category of person[a]	No. of persons (thousands)	For schizophrenia only		For schizophrenia and comorbidity		For schizophrenia and all health care spending	
		Median	Mean	Median	Mean	Median	Mean
Schizophrenia + no comorbidity	186	$3,320	$4,898	$3,320	4,898	3,949	5,990
Schizophrenia + diabetes	83	1,413	2,542	2,736	4,504	8,249	11,611
Schizophrenia + dyslipidemia	79	882	4,707	1,844	5,618	5,617	10,803
Schizophrenia + hypertension	165	1,319	2,675	1,998	3,913	8,249	12,292
Schizophrenia + heart disease	130	882	2,374	2,148	4,428	8,173	10,415

[a]Persons with more than one comorbidity appear in multiple comorbidity categories. Therefore, their expenses for total annual health care spending and spending for schizophrenia are double-counted.

From McDonald M, Hertz RP, Lustik MB, et al. Healthcare spending among community-dwelling adults with schizophrenia. *Am J Manag Care*. 2005;11(suppl):S242–S247, with permission.

Economic Analysis

Expenditures related to health care for people with diabetes are more than twice the cost of total health care without diabetes. The U.S. economy is greatly affected, with more than $92 billion spent on health care expenditures related to diabetes. In addition, indirect costs are estimated at $40 billion due to decreased productivity, lost work days, home services, permanent disability, and premature mortality.[3] Individuals with diabetes bear a disproportionate share of health care expenditures.

Health care expenditures related to comorbidities significantly increase the overall cost of treating and managing diabetes.[17] Without prevention and management of comorbid chronic conditions, costs continue to rise throughout the lifetime of individuals with diabetes. Cardiovascular disease is the most prevalent chronic condition related to diabetes mellitus and consequently it has the largest impact on cost of all chronic conditions. However, on a per capita basis, nephropathy, retinopathy, and neuropathy have higher lifetime costs.

Brandle et al. described the relationship between direct medical costs and individual demographic characteristics, treatments, glycemic control, complications, cardiovascular risk factors, and comorbidities in patients with type 2 diabetes.[18] Based on claims data, the researchers determined baseline cost through the use of median annual direct medical costs for diet-controlled diabetes with no complications or cardiovascular risk factors. Analysis of diabetes-related complications ascertained appropriate multipliers to reflect average annual costs related to treatment of complications. It may be possible to predict cost by combining baseline costs with multipliers for various conditions to determine the impact of comorbidities and treatment on direct medical costs. Conversely, the study may demonstrate reductions in cost for early intervention of risk factors and prevention of major complications. For example, patients with microalbuminuria or proteinuria have 1.17 to 1.3 times the costs for each treatment or complication, but end-stage renal failure multiples this cost by 10.53.[18] Through management of diabetes and hypertension, excessive cost related to dialysis and other medical costs, lost productivity, disability, and early mortality due to end-stage renal failure may be significantly reduced (Table 2.11).

The cost benefit of early intervention with diabetes risk factors and complications is significant both to the impact on the economy and to quality of life. Level of glycemia is a key factor in the development of complications and subsequent costs.[17] Every percentage point decrease in A_{1c} levels reduces the risk of microvascular complications such as retinopathy, neuropathy, and nephropathy by 40%.[5] However, the trend is for A_{1c} to drift upward at an average of 0.15% per year, increasing the risk of complications and costs.[17] For example, with an initial A_{1c} of 7.5%, the estimated 30-year cost is $44,145. With an initial A_{1c} of 8.0%, the cost increases to $47,943 over 30 years, and with an initial A_{1c} of 9.0%, the 30-year cost increases to $51,554.

Table **2.11**	Direct medical costs associated with demographic characteristics, treatments, diabetes complications, and comorbidities[a,b]
Disease status	**Multiplier**
Sex	
Female	1.25
BMI (kg/m^2)	
Every unit >30 kg/m^2	1.01
Diabetes intervention	
Oral antidiabetic medication	1.10
Insulin	1.59
High blood pressure	
Treated blood pressure	1.24
Retinopathy	
Nonproliferative retinopathy	—[c]
Proliferative retinopathy	—[c]
Macular edema	—[c]
Nephropathy	
Microalbuminuria	1.17
Proteinuria	1.30
ESRD with dialysis	10.53
Neuropathy	
Clinical neuropathy	—[c]
History of amputation	—[c]
Cerebrovascular disease	1.30
Cardiovascular disease	
Angina	1.73
History of myocardial infarction	1.90
Peripheral vascular disease	1.31

BMI, body mass index; ESRD = end-stage renal disease.

[a]Annual direct medical cost = baseline cost multiplied by the multiplicative factors for the combination of characteristics, treatments, and complications. In each disease category, only the multiplier associated with the most severe level of the complication should be used.

[b]The baseline cost ($1,684) represents the median annual direct medical cost for a diet-controlled white man with type 2 diabetes and BMI of 30 kg/m^2 and without microvascular, neuropathic, or cardiovascular risk factors or complications.

[c]Variables that did not enter into the model.

From Brandle M, Zhou H, Smith BRK, et al. The direct medical cost of type 2 diabetes. *Diabetes Care.* 2003;26:2300–2304, with permission.

Conversely, 30-year cost decreases by 3% if the onset of annual A_{1c} drift is delayed by 1 year. If the annual drift can be even slightly decreased, the cost savings over a 30-year period is significant. With an annual drift of 0.13%, costs decrease by 6%, and if average A_{1c} drift can be reduced by 50% to 0.075% per year, the costs are reduced by 14%.

A_{1c} levels also affect the cost of specific complications associated with diabetes. Increasing levels affect overall cost and escalate more dramatically when comorbidities are present. A_{1c} along with cardiovascular disease, hypertension, and depression are significant independent predictors of health care costs in adults with diabetes.

In addition to glycemic control, management of blood pressure reduces the risk of cardiovascular disease among people with diabetes by 33% to 50%. The risk of microvascular complications is reduced by 33% when hypertension is controlled. For every 10–mm Hg reduction in systolic blood pressure, the risk of complications related to diabetes is reduced by 12%.[5]

Preventing major complications may result in significant cost savings. For patients surviving the first year after onset, direct medical costs associated with stroke averages $26,600, acute myocardial infarction costs an average of $24,500, and amputation costs approximately $37,600.[18] Major events such as myocardial infarction, at an average cost of $30,364 per event, generate a greater financial burden than early-stage complications such as microalbuminuria, at $63 per event. However, complications that are initially relatively low in costs such as microalbuminuria can progress to more costly advanced stages such as ESRD.[63]

Treatment of level one lower-extremity ulcers has an average cost of $1,892 compared with $27,721 for amputation related to infection. Patients who progressed to higher severity levels of lower-extremity ulceration had significantly higher ulcer-related costs compared with patients who did not progress ($20,136 versus $3,063). Clearly, the high costs of treating diabetic lower-extremity ulcers emphasize the need for programs focused on preventing ulcer progression.[24]

Treatment of obesity reduces the risk of hypertension, hypercholesterolemia, coronary heart disease, stroke, and overall incidence of diabetes. Weight loss reduces the expected number of years of life with hypertension by 1.2 to 2.9 years and the expected number of years with type 2 diabetes by 0.5 to 1.7 years. For adults with a BMI greater than 27.5%, a 10% decrease in weight can reduce the lifetime risk of cardiovascular disease by 12 to 38 cases per 1,000. Furthermore, a sustained 10% reduction in body weight would decrease expected lifetime medical care costs of hypertension, hypercholesterolemia, cardiovascular disease, stroke, and type 2 diabetes by $2,200 to $5,300.[64]

The health and economic consequences of risk factors related to diabetes indicate that early intervention leading to prevention of complications saves cost related to direct medical expenditures, as well as decreases the risk of poor quality of life, disability, and premature mortality. Studies show that favorable changes in risk factors may offset at least some costs of the required treatment interventions to achieve optimal glycemic, blood pressure, and cholesterol levels.[17] Eliminating or reducing the health issues associated with diabetes through better access to preventive care, earlier diagnosis of diabetes, improved chronic disease management, and new medical technologies could greatly improve the quality of life for individuals with diabetes while reducing national expenditures for health care services and increasing productivity throughout the U.S. economy.[3]

References

1. National Health Expenditure Accounts and Average Percent Change by Type of Expenditure: Selected Calendar Years 1980–2012. CMS web site/OACT projections (cms.hhs.gov/statistics/nhe/projections-2002/t2.asp).
2. Centers for Disease Control and Prevention web site (www.cdc.gov/nccdphp).
3. Hogan P, Dall T, Nikolov P. Economic costs of diabetes in the United States in 2002. *Diabetes Care.* 2003;26:917–932.
4. Engelgau MM, Geiss LS, Saaddine JB, et al. The evolving diabetes burden in the United States. *Ann Intern Med.* 2004;140:945–950.
5. Centers for Disease Control and Prevention. National diabetes fact sheet: general information and national estimates on diabetes in the United States, 2005. Atlanta, GA: US Department of Health and Human Services, Centers for Disease Control and Prevention; 2005.
6. Cohen JW, Kraus KA, Spending and service use among people with the fifteen most costly medical conditions, 1997. *Health Aff.* 2003;22:129–138.
7. Krein S, Funnell M, Piette J. Economics of diabetes mellitus. *Nurs Clin North Am.* 2006;41:499–511.
8. American Diabetes Association. Economic consequences of diabetes mellitus in the U.S. in 1997. *Diabetes Care.* 1998;21:296–309.
9. Ng YC, Jacobs P, Johnson JA. Productivity losses associated with diabetes in the US. *Diabetes Care.* 2001;24:257–261.
10. Druss BG, Marcus SC, Olfson M, et al. The most expensive medical conditions in America. *Health Aff.* 2002;21:105–111.
11. Ramsey S, Summers KH, Leong SA, et al. Productivity and medical costs of diabetes in a large employer population. *Diabetes Care.* 2002;25:23–29.
12. Vijan S, Hayward RA, Langa KM. The impact of diabetes on workforce participation: results from a national household sample. *Health Serv Res.* 2004;39: 1653–1669.
13. U.S. Department of Health and Human Services. Healthy People 2010: Understanding and improving health. 2nd ed. Washington, DC: U.S. Government Printing Office, November 2000. www.healthypeople.gov/Document/pdf/Volume1/05Diabetes.pdf
14. Krein S, Funnell M, Piette J. Economics of diabetes mellitus. *Nurs Clin North Am.* 2006;41:499–511.
15. Geiss LA, Herman WH, Teutsch SM. Diabetes and renal mortality in the United States. *Am J Public Health.* 1985;75:1325–1326.
16. Nichols GA, Brown JB. The impact of cardiovascular disease on medical care costs in subjects with and without type 2 diabetes. *Diabetes Care.* 2002;25:482–486.

17. Caro JJ, Ward AJ, O'Brien JA. Lifetime costs of complications resulting from type 2 diabetes in the U.S. *Diabetes Care.* 2002;25:476–481.
18. Brandle M, Zhou H, Smith BRK, et al. The direct medical cost of type 2 diabetes. *Diabetes Care.* 2003;26:2300–2304.
19. Gordon A, Scuffham P, Shearer A, et al. The health care costs of diabetic peripheral neuropathy in the U.S. *Diabetes Care.* 2003;26:1790–1795.
20. Reiber GE, Boyko EJ, Smith DG. Lower extremity foot ulcers and amputations in diabetes. In: Harris M, ed. *Diabetes in America.* 2nd ed. Bethesda, MD: National Institutes of Health; 1995:409–428 (NIH publ no 95-1468).
21. Bloomgarden ZT. American Diabetes Association 60th Scientific Sessions, 2000: the diabetic foot. *Diabetes Care.* 2001;24:946–951.
22. Moss SE, Klein R, Klein BEK. Long term incidence of lower-extremity amputations in a diabetic population. *Arch Fam Med.* 1996;5:391–398.
23. Apelqvist J, Larsson J, Agardh CD. Long-term prognosis for diabetic patients with foot ulcers. *J Intern Med.* 1993;233:485–491.
24. Stockl K, Vanderplas A, Tafesse E, et al. Costs of lower-extremity ulcers among patients with diabetes. *Diabetes Care.* 2004;27:2129–2134.
25. Akbari CM, LoGerfo FW. Diabetes and peripheral vascular disease. *J Vasc Surg.* 1999;30:373–384.
26. United States Renal Data System (USRDS). USRDS 2005 Annual Data Report. Bethesda, MD: National Institute of Diabetes and Digestive and Kidney Diseases, National Institutes of Health, U.S. Department of Health and Human Services; 1998, 2001, 2003, 2005. Available at www.usrds.org.
27. Joyce AT, Iacoviello JM, Nag S, et al. End-stage renal disease—associated managed care costs among patients with and without diabetes. *Diabetes Care.* 2004;12:2829–2835.
28. National Institutes of Health, National Institute of Diabetes and Digestive and Kidney Diseases. Weight Control Information Network. Statistics Related to Overweight and Obesity. Based on data from National Health and Nutrition Examination Survey (NHANES) 2003 to 2004. http://win.niddk.nih.gov/statistica/index.htm#preval
29. National Center for Health Statistics. Chartbook on Trends in the Health of Americans. Health, United States, 2005. Hyattsville, MD: Public Health Service.
30. Flegal KM, Carroll MD, Kuczmarski RJ, et al. Overweight and obesity in the United States: Prevalence and trends, 1960–1994. *Int J Obesity.* 1998;22:39–47.
31. Clinical Guidelines on the Identification, Evaluation, and Treatment of Overweight and Obesity in Adults—The Evidence Report. National Institutes of Health. Obesity Research. 1998;6(suppl)2:51S–209S.
32. Flegal KM, Graubard BI, Williamson DF, et al. Excess deaths associated with underweight, overweight, and obesity. *JAMA.* 2005;293(15):1861–1867.
33. Fontaine KR, Redden DT, Wang C, et al. Years of life lost due to obesity. *JAMA.* 2003;289:187–193.
34. Must A, Spadano J, Coakley E, et al. The disease burden associated with overweight and obesity. *JAMA.* 1999;282:1523–1529.
35. Mokdad A, Ford ES, Bowman BA, et al. Prevalence of obesity, diabetes, and obesity-related health risk factors, 2001. *JAMA.* 2003;289:76–79.
36. Finkelstein EA, Fiebelkorn IC, Wang G. National medical spending attributable to overweight and obesity: how much and who's paying? *Health Aff.* 2003;W3:219–226.
37. The Lewin Group–American Obesity Association. Costs of obesity. 2002. http://obesity1.tempdomainname.com/treatment/cost.shtml

38. Sturm R. The effects of obesity, smoking and drinking on medical problems and costs. *Health Aff.* 2002;21:245–253.

39. Narbro K, Agren G, Jonsson E, et al. Pharmaceutical costs in obese individuals: comparison with a randomly selected population sample and long-term changes after conventional and surgical treatment: the SOS intervention study. *Arch Intern Med.* 2002;162:2061–2069.

40. Thompson D, Edelsberg J, Kinsey KL, et al. Estimated economic costs of obesity to U.S. business. *Am J Health Promot.* 1998;3:120–127.

41. Tucker LA, Friedman GM. Obesity and absenteeism: an epidemiological study of 10,825 employed adults. *Am J Health Promot.* 1998;12:202–207.

42. Wolf AM, Colditz GA. Current estimates of the economic cost of obesity in the united states. *Obes Res.* 1998;6:173–175.

43. Anderson RJ, Freedland KE, Clouse RE, et al. The prevalence of comorbid depression in adults with diabetes: a meta-analysis. *Diabetes Care.* 2001;24:1069–1078.

44. Katon WJ, von Korff M, Ciechanowski P, et al. Behavioral and clinical factors associated with depression among individuals with diabetes. *Diabetes Care.* 2004;27: 914–920.

45. Katon WJ, Rutter C, Simon G, et al. The association of comorbid depression with mortality in patients with type 2 diabetes. *Diabetes Care.* 2005;28:2668–2672.

46. Lin EHB, Katon WJ, Von Korff M, et al. Relationship of depression and diabetes self-care, medication adherence and preventive care. *Diabetes Care.* 2004;27: 2154–2160.

47. Katon WJ, Lin EHB, Russo J, et al. Cardiac risk factors in patients with diabetes mellitus and major depression. *J Gen Intern Med.* 2004;19:1192–1199.

48. Musselman DL, Betan E, Larsen H, et al. Relationship of depression to diabetes types 1 and 2: epidemiology, biology and treatment. *Biol Psychiatry.* 2003;54:317–329.

49. Joynt KE, Whellan DJ, O'Connor CM. Depression and cardiovascular disease: mechanisms of interaction. *Biol Psychiatry.* 2003;54:248–262.

50. Lustman PJ, Anderson RJ, Freedlan KE, et al. Depression and poor glycemic control: a meta-analytic review of the literature. *Diabetes Care.* 2000;23:934–942.

51. Egede LE, Nietert PJ, Zheng D. Depression and all-cause and coronary heart disease mortality among adults with and without diabetes. *Diabetes Care.* 2005;28: 1339–1345.

52. Greenberg PC, Kessler RC, Birnbaum HG, et al. The economic burden of depression in the United States: how did it change between 1999 and 2000? *J Clin Psychiatry.* 2003;64:1465–1475.

53. Egede LE, Zheng D, Simpson K. Comorbid depression is associated with increased health care use and expenditures in individuals with diabetes. *Diabetes Care.* 2002;25:464–470.

54. Ciechanowski PS, Katon WJ, Russo JE. Depression and diabetes: impact of depressive symptoms on adherence, function, and costs. *Arch Intern Med.* 2000;160: 3278–3285.

55. Finkelstein EA, Bray JW, Chen H, et al. Prevalence and costs of major depression among elderly claimants with diabetes. *Diabetes Care.* 2003;26:415–420.

56. Stewart WF, Ricci JA, Chee E, et al. Cost of lost productive work time among US workers with depression. *JAMA.* 2003;289:3135–3144.

57. Zimmet P. Epidemiology of diabetes mellitus and associated cardiovascular risk factors: focus on human immunodeficiency virus and psychiatric disorders. *Am J Med.* 2005;118(suppl 2):3S–8S.

58. Subramaniam M, Chong SA, Pek E. Diabetes mellitus and impaired glucose tolerance in patients with schizophrenia. *Can J Psychiatry.* 2003;48:345–347.
59. Kato MM, Currier MB, Gomez CM, et al. Prevalence of metabolic syndrome in Hispanic and non-Hispanic patients with schizophrenia. *Prim Care Companion J Clin Psychiatry.* 2004;6:74–77.
60. Ford ES, Giles WH, Mokdad AH. Increasing prevalence of the metabolic syndrome among US adults. *Diabetes Care.* 2004;27:2444–2449.
61. Curkendall SM, Mo J, Glasser DB, et al. Cardiovascular disease in patients with schizophrenia in Saskatchewan, Canada. *J Clin Psychiatry.* 2004;65:715–720.
62. McDonald M, Hertz RP, Lustik MB, et al. Healthcare spending among community-dwelling adults with schizophrenia. *Am J Manag Care.* 2005;11(suppl): S242–S247.
63. O'Brien JA, Patrick AR, Caro J. Estimates of direct medical costs for microvascular and macrovascular complications resulting from type 2 diabetes mellitus in the United States in 2000. *Clinical Therapeutics.* 2003;25:1017–1038.
64. Oster G, Thompson D, Edelsberg J, et al. Lifetime health and economic benefits of weight loss among obese persons. *Am J Public Health.* 1999;88:1536–1542.

CHAPTER 3

The Risk of Litigation

Jeremy M. Wilkinson

Participants in health care delivery today are in a vulnerable position. The general population has high expectations for medical management. These expectations combined with a litigious society and complex medical issues create a medicolegal minefield that professionals in the health care industry must carefully navigate. When patients suffer a negative outcome in their medical management that they believe to be caused by substandard treatment, they may file for civil damages by claiming to have suffered a *tort* (from the Latin *tortum*, meaning "wrong").[1]

When a tort is believed to have occurred by use of a particular product, the manufacturer becomes responsible for damages in what is called a *tort of product liability.*[2] Product liability is the legal avenue by which patients who experience adverse events while taking medications seek compensation for damages believed to have occurred specifically because of those medications. The defendants are often pharmaceutical companies, who manufacture and aggressively market these medications, and at times have been accused of minimizing the risk of side effects or adverse outcomes.[3] Litigation usually occurs against these large companies prior to that against individual health care personnel in hopes of potentially obtaining larger civil suit awards or settlements; it is also possible that the manufacturer had earlier awareness of a given medication's side effects.

However, as newly discovered side effects become known, the Food and Drug Administration (FDA) decides whether the benefits of a medication continue to outweigh its risks. If the product remains on the market, avoiding these dangers becomes primarily the responsibility of health care professionals trained in these matters. If substandard care is believed to have occurred in this period, the tort is often one of *malpractice* or *negligence* by the individual health care professional (e.g., physician, nurse, pharmacist).[4] For this to have occurred, four elements must be present—the four Ds:[5,6]

1. Duty (e.g., to serve, to do no harm)
2. Dereliction of duty (e.g., substandard service, avoidable harm done)
3. Damage (e.g., negative outcome)
4. Direct causation of damage (i.e., the health care provider did or did not do something that *caused* the damage)

To date, most litigation involving diabetics with mental illness has been product liability suits against manufacturers focused on a class of drugs called atypical antipsychotics or second-generation antipsychotics (SGAs), most of which entered the market after 1990. Prior to that time, antipsychotic medications (typical or first-generation antipsychotics) were the primary accepted pharmacologic option used by mental health care providers for patients suffering from psychosis. They were known to potentially cause movement disorders as a side effect from the drugs' actions on the brain, in particular *tardive dyskinesia*, a disturbing and often irreversible movement disorder. Tardive dyskinesia is characterized by repetitive and involuntary movements of the mouth and face, and at times the neck, trunk, or limbs. Until recent years, tardive dyskinesia was second only to suicide as the most frequent cause of legal action against psychiatrists.[7] As physicians transitioned their prescription habits of antipsychotic medications toward second-generation drugs, the incidence of tardive dyskinesia decreased; this is reflected in decreased numbers of tort claims filed.[7] Unfortunately, the second-generation antipsychotics have their own medicolegal risks.

The first observation of increased prevalence of metabolic derangements in schizophrenics was noted in the 1920s. Since then, it has been a widely accepted phenomenon that people afflicted with schizophrenia are more likely to become obese with hyperglycemia and abnormal lipid profiles, develop diabetes, and suffer the high-risk health problems that accompany such conditions. This has been attributed to many factors, most often to the sedentary lifestyles, smoking habits, and diets of patients, or to some undefined mechanism of glucose dysregulation associated with schizophrenia in and of itself.[8] Complicating this scenario, however, was a 2004 Consensus Panel of the American Diabetes Association, American Psychiatric Association, American Association of Clinical Endocrinologists, and North American Association for the Study of Obesity, who reported that SGAs themselves are also associated with dramatic weight gain, atherogenic lipid profiles, diabetes, and cardiovascular disease. The panel emphasized the complexity of these findings, stating the inherent prevalence of diabetes and obesity in people with schizophrenia to be approximately 1.5 to 2 times higher than that of the general population. Given this information, cause—and blame—could not be clearly demonstrated, and as such, the panel concluded only that there should be a heightened interest in the relationship between SGAs and these medical problems.[9,10] Subsequent studies have attempted to further define the roles of mental illness and SGAs in the development of metabolic derangements, but have yielded mixed or contradicting conclusions. Regardless, patients with mental illness taking SGAs for treatment were developing diabetes and experiencing other associated negative outcomes. Many believed a tort had occurred, and class action lawsuits were filed.

In the late 1990s, a series of cases were reported to the FDA suggesting olanzapine (Zyprexa, Eli Lilly and Company), risperidone (Risperdal, Janssen Pharmaceutica), clozapine (Clozaril, Novartis), and quetiapine (Seroquel, AstraZeneca) may have contributed to new-onset diabetes in patients taking these medications. Some patients died from complications, including necrotizing pancreatitis, diabetic ketoacidosis, hyperosmolar coma, and cardiovascular incidents. In 1999, in the presence of these individual claims and other academic studies, the FDA began a review to evaluate SGAs. However, the investigation was still unable to lead to definitive conclusions. Controlling bodies in Japan and the European Union already required warning labels concerning these possible complications for Zyprexa, but the FDA did not feel it a necessary step at the time in the United States.[11]

In 2001 and 2002, literature reviews of FDA reports of new-onset diabetes were conducted for Zyprexa, Risperdal, and Clozaril. In these reviews (Table 3.1), the authors found hundreds of new cases of diabetes, often with associated sequelae. The fatality rates in these patients reached upward of 8%. This is especially alarming when considering the findings were based on voluntary FDA reports, which were estimated to reflect as low as just 1% to 10% of actual events.[13] Separately, and to a lesser degree, Seroquel was reported to be associated with increased prevalence of new-onset diabetes as well.[15]

These findings and others' attempts to characterize the possible dangers of second-generation antipsychotics convinced the FDA in September 2003 to require manufacturers of SGAs to add warning statements to package inserts alerting patients and physicians to the drugs' potential risks of contributing to the onset of hyperglycemia, diabetes mellitus, ketoacidosis, hyperosmolar coma, or death.[16] By this time, two new drugs had reached the market: ziprasidone (Geodon, Pfizer) and aripiprazole (Abilify, Bristol-Myers Squibb and Otsuka America Pharmaceuticals). Aripiprazole, with a different mechanism of action than most of the other SGAs, led the entire class to become more uniformly known as atypical antipsychotic drugs. Being in the atypical antipsychotic drug class, these two new drugs were also required to insert warning labels, although they have shown—as of yet—less propensity for insulin resistance, weight gain, and metabolic side effects than their

Table **3.1**	Self-reported cases of diabetes with associated sequelae in patients on atypical antipsychotics				
Drug	**Time evaluated**	**Cases reported**	**Life-threatening**	**Fatal outcome**	**Percent fatal (%)**
Zyprexa	8 years	288	75	23	8.0
Risperdal	9 years	132	31	5	3.8
Clozaril	11 years	384	55	25	6.5

Information from Koller EA, Doraiswamy PM. Olanzapine-associated diabetes mellitus. *Pharmacotherapy.* 2002;22(7):841–852; Koller EA, Doraiswamy PM, Cross JT. Risperidone-associated diabetes. Paper presented at 84th Annual Meeting of the Endocrine Society, 2002; San Francisco, CA: 1–83; and Koller E, Schneider B, Bennett K, et al. Clozapine-associated diabetes. *Am J Med.* 2004;111(9):716–723.

predecessors, particularly olanzapine and clozapine.[17,18] Most recently, FDA approval has been granted for paliperidone (Invega, Janssen Pharmaceutica), which embeds risperidone's active metabolite in a slower-releasing matrix for ease of dosing. This drug, understandably, also warns patients and physicians of the risks of atypical antipsychotic medications.

As more studies concluded that atypical antipsychotic drugs were at least in part to blame for the side effects and negative outcomes of these widely used medications, lawsuits began to flood the legal system. In 2004, broad litigation was directed toward Eli Lilly for the effects of patients taking Zyprexa. In April 2004, pending lawsuits were so plentiful and geographically dispersed that many were joined into a large class action lawsuit. The plaintiffs argued that Eli Lilly did not sufficiently warn patients or physicians of the potential risks of developing hyperglycemia and/or diabetes prior to September 2003. In June 2005, the manufacturer agreed to settle this class action lawsuit for $690 million, resolving an estimated 8,000 claims, thought to represent about 75% of existing lawsuits.[19] However, this settlement, combined with further research and greater public awareness, led to even more claims. In January 2007, another 18,000 lawsuits were settled by Eli Lilly for approximately $500 million for similar complaints. Included in the agreement was release of liability (i.e., torts of negligence or malpractice) directed toward physicians for the prescription of Zyprexa prior to September 2003.[20] Troubles for Eli Lilly are likely to continue, because a December 2006 article in the *New York Times* alleges that the drug manufacturer has long acknowledged internally—and kept private—data linking Zyprexa to obesity and hyperglycemia.[3]

Even prior to the onset of the Zyprexa lawsuits, litigation was filed against the makers of Seroquel for similar claims of inadequate warnings on medication labels. Although data for Seroquel were less convincing, and it is prescribed less frequently than olanzapine, this litigation has been slower to move through the legal system and is comprised mostly of class action and mass tort suits. These lawsuits began to take shape in August 2003 and have been aggressively recruiting patients who have taken the medication, as has become the case with each atypical antipsychotic drug. As of February 2007, AstraZeneca acknowledged the existence of more than 1200 lawsuits representing more than 8,000 patients.[21]

Although to date, Eli Lilly is the only manufacturer to pay significant financial penalty for the side effects experienced by patients taking its medication, it is clear that Astrazeneca faces similar concerns in the near future. The manufacturers of each of the other atypical antipsychotics also potentially face significant risk in the upcoming years. A simple Internet search yields abundant law firms seeking potential plaintiffs for large civil suits against manufacturers for each atypical antipsychotic drug.

Data is still inconclusive about direct causality of these medications, but awareness is such that individual health care professionals are now responsible for helping patients navigate these risks. These professionals who focus primarily on improved mental health must now show greater diligence in protecting their patients' physical health as well. This requires improved communication and awareness of potential dangers; regular monitoring of glucose, weight, and lipid panels; side effect prevention; detailed documentation; vigorous attempts to stay current with new information and guidelines; and—when necessary—partnering with professionals of other disciplines better trained in prevention of specific side effects and their sequelae.[7] There is great risk of litigation in the complicated medicolegal world of diabetes in the mentally ill. The best way to prevent legal recourse is to avoid negative outcomes in the first place, an immense challenge requiring health care personnel to be proactive and dedicated to providing the highest level of patient care.

References

1. *Crystal Reference Encyclopedia.* Tort definition. http://encyclopedia.jrank. org/Cambridge/entries/080/tort.html. Accessed March 25, 2007.
2. Black HC, Connolly MJ, Nolan JR. *Black's Law Dictionary.* 5th ed. St. Paul, MN: West Publishing; 1979: 1089.
3. Berenson, Alex. Eli Lilly said to play down risk of top pill. *New York Times,* December 17, 2006:Page 1.1. www.nytimes.com/2006/12/17/business/17drug. html. Accessed March 25, 2007.
4. *The Columbia Electronic Encyclopedia.* 6th ed. Columbia University Press. 2003. Tort of malpractice and negligence definition. http://www. answers.com/topic/ malpractice#copyright. Accessed March 25, 2007.
5. Prosser, W. L. *Handbook of the Law of Torts.* 4th ed. St. Paul, MN: West Publishing, 1971.
6. Rothblatt HB, Leroy, DH. Avoiding psychiatric malpractice. *California West Law Rev.* 1973;(9):260–272.
7. Wirshing D, Wirshing W, Nystrom M, et al. Medicolegal considerations in the treatment of psychosis with second-generation antipsychotics. *Psychiatr Times.* 2004;21(14). www.psychiatrictimes.com/showarticle.jhtml?articleID= 59100055. Accessed March 25, 2007.
8. "Schizophrenia and Diabetes 2003" Expert Consensus Meeting, Dublin, 3–4 October 2003, Consensus summary. *B J Psychiatry.* 2004;184(suppl 47):s112–s114.
9. Kaplan A. Consensus panel urges monitoring for metabolic effects of atypical antipsychotics. *Psychiatr Times,.*2004;21(4). www.psychiatrictimes.com/p04041B. htm. Accessed March 25, 2007.
10. American Diabetes Association, American Psychiatric Association, American Association of Clinical Endocrinologists, North American Association for the Study of Obesity. Consensus development conference on antipsychotic drugs and obesity and diabetes. *Diabetes Care.* 2004;27(2):596–601.
11. Anand G, Burton TM. Drug debate: new antipsychotics pose a quandary for FDA, doctors—Eli Lilly's big seller, Zyprexa, can help schizophrenics; is it linked to diabetes?— warnings abroad, not in U.S. *Wall Street Journal.* April 11, 2003;241:A1, A8.
12. Koller EA, Doraiswamy PM. Olanzapine-associated diabetes mellitus. *Pharmacotherapy.* 2002;22(7):841–852.
13. Koller EA, Doraiswamy PM, Cross JT. Risperidone-associated diabetes. Paper presented at 84th Annual Meeting of the Endocrine Society, 2002; San Francisco, CA: 1–83.

14. Koller E, Schneider B, Bennett K, et al. Clozapine-associated diabetes. *Am J Med.* 2004;111(9):716–723.
15. Sernyak MJ, Leslie DL, Alarcon RD, et al. Association of diabetes mellitus with use of atypical neuroleptics in the treatment of schizophrenia. *Am J Psychiatry.* 2002;159:561–566.
16. FDA's proposed diabetes warning. *Psychiatr News.* 2003;38(20):26.
17. Melkersson K, Dahl M-L. Adverse metabolic effects associated with atypical antipsychotics: literature review and clinical implications. *Drugs.* 2004;64 (7):701–723.
18. Nasrallah HA, Newcomer JW. Atypical antipsychotics and metabolic dysregulation: evaluating the risk/benefit equation and improving the standard of care. *J Clin Psychopharmacol.* 2004;24(5 suppl 1):S7–S14.
19. Legal News Watch. Lilly agrees to pay $690M to settle Zyprexa class action lawsuits. http://www.legalnewswatch.com. June 15, 2005. Accessed on yyyy #, zzzzz. Accessed March 25, 2007.
20. *Legal News Watch.* Zyprexa lawsuits: Lilly agrees to settle most claims. 5 Jan 2007. http://www.legalnewswatch.com:. Accessed March 25, 2007.
21. Fisk, Margaret C. AstraZeneca faces 10,000 lawsuits over Seroquel drug. 13 Feb 2007. http://www.bloomberg.com/apps/news?pid=20601102&sid=a.ZTdmV67chI &refer=uk. Accessed March 25, 2007.

Psychotropic Medications and Metabolic Disorders

*Cara F. Adamson Greene
and Jennifer A. Rosen*

Many medications, in particular psychotropics, including antidepressants, antipsychotics, and mood stabilizers, are associated with elevations in blood pressure, weight gain, dyslipidemias, and/or impaired glucose homeostasis. It is clear that the prevalence of diabetes and its risk factors is much greater in patients with serious mental illness, particularly in patients with schizophrenia. Studies have found the prevalence of both diabetes and obesity to be two to four times higher in people with schizophrenia than in the general population, with an overall prevalence estimate of 12% for diabetes in patients with schizophrenia.[1]

Medications contributing to the development of metabolic syndrome through obesity, impaired glucose homeostasis, diabetes, and dyslipidemia are of important concern when treating this particular patient population. These patients are at higher cardiovascular and metabolic risk to begin with, due in part to a variety of causes including profound negative symptoms, cognitive disorganization, lack of access or financial means for healthier food options, and an increased prevalence of smoking. Various psychotropics have been associated with weight gain and impaired glucose homeostasis, and the atypical antipsychotics in particular have been associated with insulin resistance and the metabolic syndrome.

Figure 4.1 illustrates the potential sites at which medication may induce changes in glucose metabolism. A number of medications, which will not be discussed in detail, are also associated with hypoglycemia. Table 4.1 serves as a review of these agents

Antidepressants

Patients with major depression have symptoms that reflect changes in brain monoamine neurotransmitters, specifically norepinephrine (NE), serotonin (5-HT), and dopamine. Antidepressants act on these neurotransmitter pathways and are classified based on established pharmacology.

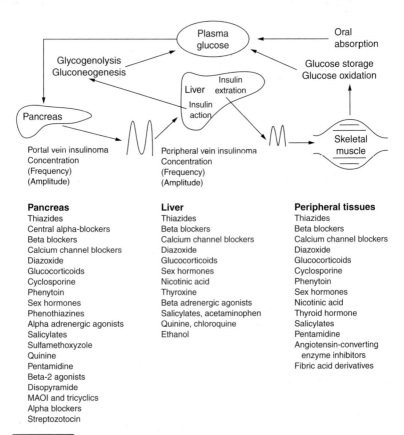

To date, no prospective study has directly compared the efficacy and tolerability of selective serotonin reuptake inhibitors (SSRIs), serotonin/norepinephrine reuptake inhibitors (SNRIs), or other second-generation antidepressants in patients with diabetes versus patients without diabetes. Table 4.2 summarizes the effects of antidepressants on body weight. Table 4.3 summarizes the effects of newer antidepressants on blood glucose.

| Table **4.1** | Medications/drugs associated with hypoglycemia |

Antibacterials
Isoniazid
Gatifloxacin
Levofloxacin
Pentamidine
Sulfonamides or sulfa drugs
Trimethoprim
Antidepressants
Tricyclics
Fluoxetine
Sertraline
Antidiabetic agents
Oral hypoglycemics
Insulin
Antihypertensives
Angiotensin-converting enzyme inhibitors
Propranolol (plus ethanol)
Thiazide diuretics
Antipsychotics
Chlorpromazine
Haloperidol
Antiretrovirals
Didanosine
Chemotherapy Agents
Cytotoxic agents
6-Mercaptopurine
Methotrexate
Phenylbutazone
Cholesterol lowering agents
Clofibrate
Nonsteroidal anti-inflammatories
Salicylates
Mood stabilizers
Lithium
Others
Disopyramide
Ethanol
Propoxyphene
Quinidine
Quinine
Ritodrine
Stanozolol

Data from Pandit MK, Burke J, Gustafson AB, et al. Drug-induced disorders of glucose tolerance. *Ann Intern Med.* 1993;118 (7):529–539 and Guettier JM. Hypoglycemia. *Endocrinol Metab Clin North Am.* 2006;35(4):753–766.

Table **4.2**	Effects of antidepressants on body weight
Antidepressant	**Effect on weight**
Bupropion	Likely to cause weight loss
Monoamine oxidase inhibitors (MAOIs)	Weight gain likely in short term (<6 months) and long term (≥1 year)
Selective serotonin reuptake inhibitors (SSRIs) other than paroxetine	Weight gain in short term less likely. Weight gain in long term possible, but evidence is varied
Mirtazapine	More likely than placebo to cause weight gain in short term, but less likely than TCAs
Nefazodone	Likely to have no effect on weight
Paroxetine	Weight gain in short and long terms more likely than for other SSRIs
Tricyclic antidepressants (TCAs)	Weight gain likely in short term and long term
Venlafaxine	Likely to have no effect on weight

From Deshmukh R, Franco K. Managing weight gain as a side effect of antidepressant therapy. *Cleve Clin J Med.* 2003;70(7):614–623. http://www.ccjm.org/pdffiles/Deshmuhk703.pdf, with permission.

Table **4.3**	Effects of antidepressants on glucose	
Antidepressant	**Effect on glucose**	**Clinical significance**
Citalopram[112]	Decrease or increase	Unknown
Fluoxetine[110, 111]	Decrease	Low to moderate
Maprotiline[105]	Decrease	Moderate to high
Nefazodone[104,109]	Decrease	High (has caused hypoglycemia attacks in one stabilized diabetic patient)
Paroxetine[106]	Decrease or increase	Unknown
Selegiline[19,103,108]	Decrease	High
Sertraline[107,110]	Decrease	Low to moderate (has induced serious hypoglycemia in one nondiabetic patient)
TCAs[5]	Increase	Low to moderate

Tricyclic Antidepressants: The tricyclic antidepressants (TCAs) are effective in treating all depressive subtypes. TCAs potentiate the activity of NE and 5-HT by blocking their reuptake. However, the potency and selectivity of the TCAs for the inhibition of NE and 5-HT vary. Because TCAs affect other receptor systems, anticholinergic, neurologic, and cardiovascular adverse events are frequently reported during TCA therapy. The most common side effects associated with TCAs are dry mouth, constipation, blurred vision, urinary retention, dizziness, tachycardia, memory impairment, and, at higher doses, delirium. These effects may result from blockade of cholinergic receptors. A common and potentially serious side effect of the TCAs is orthostatic hypotension. TCAs also cause cardiac conduction delays and may even induce heart block in patients with pre-existing conduction disease.

Effects on Weight Weight is a common and well-known adverse effect of short-term and long-term treatment with TCAs, primarily as a result of excessive appetite.[2] Possible mechanisms include blockade of histamine-1 (H_1) and serotonin 2C (5HT-2c) receptors, carbohydrate craving caused by alpha-noradrenergic activity or histamine blockade, changes in the regulation of body fat stores by modulating neurotransmitter systems at the hypothalamic level, and recovery from clinical depression.[2] Because tertiary TCAs, such as amitriptyline, imipramine, and doxepin, are stronger histamine blockers than are secondary tricyclics such as desipramine and nortriptyline, the tertiary tricyclic drugs, amitriptyline in particular, are more likely to cause weight gain.[2,3] Interestingly, weight gain is the most common cause for premature discontinuation of all TCAs.[4]

Effects on Glucose TCAs are more likely to impair diabetes control, because they increase serum glucose levels by up to 150%, increase appetite (particularly carbohydrate craving), and reduce the metabolic rate.[5] They are generally considered safe in patients with diabetes, unless the diabetes is very poorly controlled or the patient suffers from significant cardiac or renal disease.

Serotonin/Norepinephrine Reuptake Inhibitors: Venlafaxine is a potent inhibitor of 5-HT and NE reuptake and weak inhibitor of dopamine reuptake. Unlike the TCAs, it has virtually no affinity for muscarinic, histaminergic, or alpha-adrenergic receptors. The most commonly reported side effects with venlafaxine include nausea, constipation, somnolence, dry mouth, dizziness, nervousness, sweating, asthenia, abnormal ejaculation/orgasm, anorexia, and increases in blood pressure. Side effects are dose-related.

Duloxetine is also a potent inhibitor of 5-HT and NE reuptake and weak inhibitor of dopamine reuptake, but it has not been associated with increases in blood pressure. It is Food and Drug Administration (FDA)–approved for major depressive disorder and diabetic peripheral neuropathic pain.

Effects on Blood Pressure Venlafaxine may cause a dose-related increase in diastolic blood pressure. Interestingly, baseline blood pressure is not a useful predictor of the occurrence of this phenomenon. In placebo-controlled studies, clinically significant increases in blood pressure (increase in diastolic blood pressure of ≥ 15 mm Hg and to ≥ 105 mm Hg from baseline) were observed in 5.5% of patients at doses greater than 200 mg daily. The mean increase in diastolic blood pressure was 7 mm Hg after 6 weeks of treatment with doses of 300 to 375 mg daily.[6] In comparative trials, the overall incidence of clinically significant blood pressure increases with venlafaxine was similar to that of TCAs.[6]

Effects on Weight A short-term study comparing venlafaxine with fluoxetine found no significant weight gain with venlafaxine.[7] Similarly, duloxetine, a newer agent, has not been associated with weight gain.

Atypical Antidepressants: Trazodone and nefazodone are members of the triazolopyridine class. Both have dual actions on serotonergic neurons acting as both a 5-H_{2c} receptor antagonist and 5-HT reuptake inhibitor, and they appear to enhance 5-HT1a-mediated neurotransmission. These drugs have negligible affinity for cholinergic and histaminergic receptors. Nefazodone also has low affinity for alpha$_1$-adrenergic receptors. Both agents can cause orthostatic hypotension. Sedation and cognitive slowing are the most frequent dose-limiting side effects associated with trazodone. Trazodone has been associated with a rare but potentially serious side effect priapism (occurs in 1 in 6,000 patients).[8] Common side effects for nefazodone include lightheadedness, dizziness, orthostatic hypotension, somnolence, dry mouth, nausea, and asthenia. Nefazodone, manufactured as Serzone, was voluntarily removed from U.S. markets in 2004 amid concerns of hepatotoxicity resulting in liver failure or death (one reported case per 250,000 to 300,000 patient-years).[9] Generic formulations of nefazodone are still available.

Effects on Weight A 36-week placebo-controlled study reported weight associated with nefazodone to be similar to placebo (7.6% vs. 8.6%).[10] Sussman et al. conducted a pooled analysis of three clinical trials comparing nefazodone with SSRIs and three clinical trials comparing nefazodone with imipramine. Using a 7% or greater weight change as a measure of clinical significance, results indicated that 4.3% of SSRI-treated patients had lost weight at some point in the acute phase of the trial (6 to 8 weeks) versus 1.7% with nefazodone. During longer treatment (16 to 46 weeks), weight gain occurred more often in patients taking an SSRI compared with patients taking nefazodone (17.9% vs. 8.3%). Patients taking imipramine also had a greater increase in body weight than patients taking nefazodone in both short-term and long-term phases, indicating that nefazodone may be less likely to cause weight gain than both SSRIs and TCAs when used longer than 1 year.[11]

Bupropion: Bupropion is a novel antidepressant with a unique mechanism of action. It has no appreciable effect on the reuptake of 5-HT, and its most potent neurochemical action is blockade of dopamine reuptake. It is essentially devoid of antihistaminic effects and has commonly been associated with weight loss. Adverse effects associated with bupropion include nausea, dizziness, tremor, insomnia, vomiting, constipation, dry mouth, and skin reactions. The occurrence of seizures in patients taking bupropion appears to be strongly correlated with higher doses and may be increased by predisposing factors such as history of head trauma and or the presence of a tumor in the central nervous system. At daily doses of 300 to 450 mg/day, the incidence of seizures is 0.4%. At 600 mg/day, the incidence is 2.3% and at doses between 600 and 900 mg/day, seizures occur in 2.8% of patients.

Effects on Weight In a 52-week acute and continuation trial, bupropion was associated with a moderate loss of body weight (–1.15 kg from baseline).[12]

Mirtazapine: Mirtazapine is believed to enhance central noradrenergic and serotonergic activity as a 5-HT2 and 5-HT3 receptor antagonist. Mirtazapine has been associated with increases in cholesterol as well as weight gain.

Effects on Weight Across comparative trials, mirtazapine was associated with an approximate mean incidence of weight gain of 13%. Two randomized studies assessing the efficacies of mirtazapine and paroxetine reported significantly greater weight gain in the mirtazapine group than in the paroxetine group.[13,14] The weight gain associated with mirtazapine may be due to its activity at histamine receptors. In a long-term continuation of a trial of acute treatment, patients continued treatment with mirtazapine, amitriptyline, or placebo for up to 2 years.[15] Weight gain was more common with amitriptyline (22%) than mirtazapine (13%), but significantly more patients taking mirtazapine experienced weight gain than those taking the placebo. A comparison of mirtazapine and venlafaxine in the treatment of severely depressed hospitalized patients with melancholic features identified a significant weight gain of 2.0 ± 3.7 kg in the mirtazapine group and a loss of 0.5 ± 2.9 kg in the venlafaxine group.[16]

Effects on Lipids In premarketing trials, nonfasting cholesterol levels increased to 20% or more above the upper limits of normal in 15% of patients treated with mirtazapine.[17] Furthermore, in a 4-week study of healthy subjects, those treated with mirtazapine experienced a significant increase in body weight from baseline (mean increase 3.64 lb), suggesting that the weight gain caused by mirtazapine is independent of the weight changes associated with recovering depression.[18] This trial also quantified the changes in total cholesterol low-density lipoprotein (LDL) cholesterol, and triglycerides associated with mirtazapine treatment. After 4 weeks of therapy, mirtazapine-treated subjects experienced a significant increase in total cholesterol (mean increase 7.6 mg/dL) and nonsignificant increases in LDL cholesterol and triglyceride levels compared to baseline, whereas no significant changes were noted in placebo-treated patients. Among treated patients, weight increase was linearly associated with increasing total cholesterol. The results of this short-term trial have suggested that weight and cholesterol changes associated with mirtazapine occur independently of depression recovery.

Monoamine Oxidase Inhibitors: Monoamine oxidase inhibitors (MAOIs) increase the concentrations of NE, 5-HT, and dopamine within the neuronal synapse through inhibition of the monoamine oxidase enzyme and are believed to be most useful in atypical depression (symptoms that include mood reactivity, irritability, hypersomnia, hyperphagia, and psychomotor agitation). The most common adverse effect of MAOIs is postural hypotension, which is more significant with phenelzine than tranylcypromine. Anticholinergic side effects, especially dry mouth and constipation, are common but are mild compared with those associated with the TCAs. Hypertensive crisis, a potentially fatal but rare adverse reaction occurs when MAOIs are taken concurrently with certain drugs or foods, especially those high in tyramine; this dangerous side effect has limited the use of MAOIs despite their great efficacy. Education of patients taking MAOIs regarding dietary and medication restrictions is extremely important.

EMSAM is a newer MAOI released in 2006. It is a transdermal selegiline formulation. Selegiline is also available in an oral formulation at lower doses for the treatment of Parkinson's disease. At lower doses, selegiline selectively inhibits monoamine oxidase -B, however, at higher concentrations necessary to treat depression, selegiline inhibits both monoamine oxidase -B and monoamine oxidase -A. The monoamine oxidase enzyme in the gastrointestinal tract and liver (primarily type A), for example, is thought to provide vital protection from exogenous amines (e.g., tyramine) that have the capacity, if absorbed intact, to cause a "hypertensive crisis," the so-called "cheese reaction." At higher doses, EMSAM carries similar dietary warnings to other MAOI antidepressants.

Effects on Weight Of the MAOIs, phenelzine has been most associated with weight gain; however, this conclusion is based primarily on case reports. Another MAOI, tranylcypromine, may cause weight loss due to structural similarities to amphetamines.[19] Among adverse events reported with EMSAM, weight loss was more common than weight gain.[20]

Effects on Glucose The effect of MAOIs on glucose is unclear. The hydrazine group of MAOIs can cause hypoglycemia due to direct stimulation of insulin release and can also potentiate hypoglycemia. Mebanazine appears particularly likely to result in hypoglycemia, and this effect can last for several weeks. However, the increase in dopamine and norepinephrine associated with MAOIs may actually result in hyperglycemia.[21]

Selective Serotonin Reuptake Inhibitors: As the name implies, SSRIs work by inhibiting the reuptake of serotonin. In general, the SSRIs have a low affinity for histamine, alpha-adrenergic, and muscarinic receptors. They produce fewer anticholinergic and cardiovascular adverse effects than the TCAs. Some adverse effects are generally mild and short-lived, such as gastrointestinal symptoms (nausea, vomiting, diarrhea) and possible increased anxiety. Headache, insomnia, and fatigue are commonly reported. In addition, sexual dysfunction has been reported in both males and females.

Effects on Weight In clinical trials, SSRIs have been associated with both weight gain and weight loss. Weight change induced by SSRIs is likely related to alteration in 5HT2c receptor activity, appetite increase, carbohydrate craving, or recovery from clinical depression.[2] Weight gain is less likely with SSRIs when they are used short term—for 6 months or less. Contradictory evidence exists about whether an increase in body weight occurs in patients using SSRIs for 1 year or longer. In its practice guideline for the treatment of major depressive disorder, the American Psychiatric Association (APA) acknowledges that the literature differs as to whether patients taking SSRIs beyond the acute phase experience weight gain as a medication side effect.[22]

The mean incidence of weight gain across comparative randomized controlled trials ranges from 4.1% for fluoxetine, 7.6% for sertraline, and 9.6% for paroxetine.[23] A 32-week acute and continuation trial assessed differences in weight changes among patients treated with fluoxetine, paroxetine, and sertraline. Paroxetine patients showed a significantly greater mean weight change ($+3.6\%$) than did those taking fluoxetine (-0.2%; $p = 0.015$) and sertraline ($+1.0\%$; $p < 0.001$). Significantly more patients in the paroxetine group (25.5%) had a weight gain of more than seven percent than in the fluoxetine (6.8%; $p = 0.016$) and sertraline groups (4.2%; $p = 0.003$).[24] An open-label, nonrandomized, 2.5-year study in patients with obsessive-compulsive disorder also reported the lowest increase in weight gain for fluoxetine ($+0.5$ kg). Other SSRIs have led to greater weight gains (sertraline $+1.0$ kg; citalopram $+1.5$ kg; paroxetine $+1.7$ kg; fluvoxamine $+1.7$ kg); however, differences were neither statistically nor clinically significant.[25] Paroxetine may be more likely than other SSRIs to cause weight gain during short-term or long-term treatment.[2]

Effects on Glucose SSRIs may reduce serum glucose by up to 30% and cause appetite suppression, resulting in weight loss. Fluoxetine should be used cautiously in patients with diabetes, because of its increased potential for hypoglycemia, particularly in non–insulin-dependent diabetes. Its side effects of tremor, nausea, sweating, and anxiety may also be misinterpreted as due to hypoglycemia.[26] If fluoxetine is prescribed for a patient with diabetes, the patient should be advised of the need to monitor serum glucose levels regularly.

Antipsychotics

The first-generation antipsychotic medications available on the market, typical antipsychotics, were dopaminergic antagonists. Among these compounds, there are differences in their affinities for D1 and D2 receptors; however, these differences do not appear to be clinically significant.

Prior to the development of the second-generation antipsychotics (SGAs), or atypical antipsychotics, phenothiazines were the dominant therapy for schizophrenia. Numerous studies at this time began documenting that the use of phenothiazines led to aggravation of preexisting diabetes and the development of new-onset type 2 diabetes. Early reports suggested that phenothiazines cause increased insulin resistance, and this impression was supported by the fact that chlorpromazine was used successfully in the treatment of malignant insulinoma. Interestingly, the association between phenothiazines and hyperglycemia was not reported equally for all of the first-generation antipsychotics. The high-potency neuroleptics, in particular (i.e., haloperidol), appeared to be less implicated in the development of diabetes. These drugs eventually became the predominant form of therapy for schizophrenia, and the number of reports of hyperglycemia and antipsychotics subsequently dropped dramatically.

Unfortunately, the high-potency neuroleptics are also associated with a high rate of occurrence of extrapyramidal symptoms, tardive dyskinesia, and subsequent noncompliance with medications. In the late 1980s, a new class of antipsychotics, the thiobenzodiazepines or "atypical antipsychotics," was introduced. Clozapine was the first drug in this class that was widely used in North America. One major advantage of these agents was a marked reduction in the occurrence of extrapyramidal symptoms. Importantly, these drugs also proved to be clinically superior for treating schizophrenia and at reducing negative symptoms. Moreover, many of the SGAs have proven superior in reducing rates of depression and suicide, improving cognition, and improving overall quality of life. This latter attribute is particularly true of clozapine, which has recently been approved by the FDA to decrease the risk of suicide.

However, the atypical antipsychotics have also proven to carry their own unique side-effect profile. Side effects include substantial weight gain, which can also be associated with some of the classical neuroleptics, but which appears to be even more common with the SGAs. Additionally, lipid abnormalities, including elevations in triglycerides, have been reported. Hyperglycemia and diabetes are strongly associated with some of the newer atypical antipsychotics as well. Thus, many psychiatrists are finding themselves in the difficult position of trading efficacy in the treatment of schizophrenia for an array of adverse metabolic side effects.

Atypical Antipsychotics: Atypical is the term applied to antipsychotic neuroleptics that produce few or no extrapyramidal symptoms and potentially have clinical response patterns different than traditional antipsychotics. More recently, the atypical antipsychotics are becoming known as SGAs. The mechanism of action of the SGAs differs among drugs in this class. The SGAs work as antagonists at various receptor sites, including various dopamine and histamine receptors, as well as muscarinic receptors, H_1 receptors, and alpha$_1$ receptors.

Metabolic Effects and the Metabolic Syndrome: The SGAs have been associated with metabolic effects to a varying degree. Certain SGAs have been reported to produce substantial weight gain and an increased risk of dyslipidemia and type 2 diabetes. The classic triad of the metabolic syndrome are weight gain, diabetes, and dyslipidemia These physical findings, in turn, cause an array of problems—most notably cardiovascular disease (CVD) and the end products of diabetes (i.e., retinopathy, renal disease, neuropathy, and in severe cases, amputations).

Obesity and type 2 diabetes have been described as an epidemic in America and both are more prominent among people taking atypical antipsychotics.[27] An American Diabetes Association (ADA) consensus development report, cosponsored by the American Psychiatric Association (APA), the American Association of Clinical Endocrinologists, and the North American Association for the Study of Obesity, noted that among SGAs, clozapine and olanzapine are associated with the greatest potential for weight gain, as well as an increased risk of type 2 diabetes and dyslipidemia.[28] Clozapine and olanzapine are followed by risperidone and quetiapine, in terms of their effects on weight, glucose, and lipids. Although limited comparative and limited long-term data are available, ziprasidone and aripiprazole appear to carry the lowest risk of metabolic abnormalities amongst the atypical agents. The report emphasized that physicians should consider multiple factors, including the presence of medical and psychiatric conditions, when evaluating the risks and benefits of prescribing specific antipsychotic agents, and that the potential benefits of prescribing specific antipsychotics with metabolic liabilities might, under certain circumstances, outweigh the potential risks.

Effects on Weight Weight gain is one of the more noticeable effects of all of the psychotropics. Although the SGAs appear to be a major culprit, TCAs, lithium, and mood stabilizers such as valproic acid or divalproex sodium and carbamazepine are also associated with weight gain.

Although weight gain can develop over the entire body, abdominal obesity is of most concern. Increases in abdominal girth are associated with a number of negative outcomes including dyslipidemia, and a higher risk of diabetes and CVD. Abdominal circumferences over 40 inches in a man or over 35 inches in a woman in conjunction with other factors is linked to metabolic syndrome.[29] Kawachi[30] looked at the lessons taught of Nurses' Health Study and came to these conclusions:

1. A complex relationship exists between weight change since age 18 and total mortality.
2. Weight gain of a modest one pound per year from age 18 was associated with premature death.

3. A weight gain of 44 pounds was significantly correlated to high mortality.
4. A weight gain of 11 pounds increased the risk of CVD.
5. The more weight gained, the greater the risk of CVD.
6. A linear relationship exists between weight gain and hypertension.
7. An exponential relationship exists between weight gain and type 2 diabetes. To meet the criteria for metabolic syndrome, one must possess three of the following risk factors: (a) increased abdominal girth, (b) elevated triglycerides, (c) low high-density lipoprotein (HDL) cholesterol, (d) elevated blood pressure, or (e) elevated fasting glucose (Table 4.4). Because obesity and weight gain are major risk factors for insulin resistance and type 2 diabetes, weight gain associated with the SGAs is extremely concerning, because this further compounds the risk of developing metabolic syndrome.

A review of absolute weight gain in various placebo-controlled trials and head-to-head comparisons found that the relative incidence and magnitude of weight gain was not equal among antipsychotic medications.[31] Short-term treatment with various agents has been reported to produce an increase body weight ranging from less than one killogram to slightly greater than four killograms.[32,33] However, studies of the long-term effects of the SGAs on weight are more relevant to clinical practice. When multiple doses assessed in the clinical trial programs are pooled, aripiprazole and ziprasidone are associated with a mean weight gain of about 1 kg over 1 year; quetiapine and risperidone with a gain of 2 to 3 kg over 1 year; and olanzapine with a gain of more than 10 kg, which was observed in patients who received olanzapine at daily doses between 12.5 and 17.5 mg, the highest doses tested in large-scale pivotal trials.[34,35] Among the comparative studies, a higher proportion of patients experienced weight gain with olanzapine compared to risperidone.

The Clinical Antipsychotic Trials in Intervention Effectiveness (CATIE) study, a major prospective trial sponsored by the U.S. National Institutes of

Table **4.4**	Major physical findings associated with metabolic syndrome
Three or more of the following constitute the "metabolic syndrome"	
Waist size	> 40 inches in men or >35 inches in women
Elevated triglycerides	≥150 mg/dL[a]
Low high-density lipid cholesterol	< 40 mg/dL in men or <50 mg/dL in women[a]
Elevated blood pressure	≥130/85 mm Hg[a]
Elevated fasting glucose	≥100 mg/dL[a]

[a]Or taking medication for this factor.
Adapted from Grundy SM. Metabolic syndrome scientific statement by the American Heart Association and the National Heart, Lung, and Blood Institute. *Arterioscl Thromb Vas Biol.* 2005;24:2243–2244.

Mental Health, was designed to assess the efficacy of the SGAs, including olanzapine, quetiapine, risperidone, and ziprasidone, with perphenazine included as a first-generation agent.[36] The trial included 1,493 patients with schizophrenia from 57 sites in the United States. The primary outcome measure was time to all-cause discontinuation. Secondary outcome measures included assessment of the reasons for discontinuation (for example, lack of efficacy compared with intolerability owing to side effects, the latter including weight gain and metabolic disturbances).

Phase I results of the CATIE study were published in September 2005. Olanzapine was found to be more effective than the other agents in terms of discontinuation rates; however, there was an alarmingly high discontinuation rate of 74% for all treatments. Patients in the olanzapine group gained more weight than patients in any other group (mean weight gain of 0.9 kg monthly), and 30% of patients in the olanzapine group gained 7% or more of their baseline body weight (compared with 7% to 16% in the other groups, $p < 0.001$).

In a pooled analysis of four comparative studies between olanzapine and risperidone, the relative risk of weight gain was higher with olanzapine than with risperidone (2.47, 95% confidence interval [CI] 1.65–3.70). The weighted mean weight gain was 1.8 kg higher (95% CI 0.49–3.11).[37]

In a safety and tolerability 26-week study, 37% of olanzapine-treated patients versus 14% of aripiprazole-treated patients experienced a weight gain of ≥7% increase from baseline ($p < 0.01$). Both treatment groups achieved comparable improvement on efficacy measures.[38]

Two uncontrolled, open-label studies reported long-term weight changes with risperidone treatment in children with autism. In a study of primarily children and widely varying degrees of mental functioning, mean doses were 2.5 mg/day at 6 months (n = 11) and 2.7 mg/day at 12 months (n = 7). The mean age in this study was 12.6 years (range 7 to 17). The other study also primarily included patients diagnosed with autism and a wide range of mental function but required that the patients had severe aggressive symptoms. The mean dose in this study was 1.8 mg/day during a 16-week acute phase and 2.4 mg/day during the 24-week maintenance phase. In both, average gain was about 4 kg at 6 months. In one, the gain continued through 12 months at about the same rate (average gain 8.2 kg at 12 months); whereas in the other it slowed after 6 months (average gain 3.3 kg from 6 to 12 months.).[37]

It has also been reported that the risk of weight gain is increased in antipsychotic-naïve patients, and weight gain itself may not be dose dependent.[39] Table 4.5 summarizes several studies of the effects of SGAs on weight.

Effects on Glucose Diabetes occurs more often in people with schizophrenia than in the general population. This was true even before the advent of antipsychotics.[27] Diabetes is known to lead to organ damage, blindness, renal failure, and amputations. Clozapine and olanzapine are the agents most

Table **4.5**	Mean weight gain in observational studies of atypical antipsychotics		
Study	N	Duration	Mean weight increase (kg)
Olanzapine			
Littrell 2001	30	1 year	7.7
Kinon 2001 (olanzapine arm)	573	2.6 years	6.26
Sanger 2001	113	6.6 months	6.64
Quetiapine			
Tairot 2000	184	8.4 months	0.3
Brecher 2000	427	1 year	1.94
Risperidone			
Moller 1998	386	Up to ~1 year	1.8

From McDonagh MS, Peterson K, Carson S. Drug class review on atypical antipsychotic drugs. Final Report April 2006. Oregon Health & Science University Evidence-based Practice Center. http://www.ohsu.edu/drugeffectiveness/reports/documents/AAPs%20Final%20Report%20Update%201.pdf. Accessed September 10, 2007, with permission.

closely coupled to diabetes, whereas aripiprazole and ziprasidone show less likelihood of precipitating the disorder.[40] Obesity contributes to diabetes due to its associated hyperglycemia, dyslipidemia, and insulin resistance. Although the exact meaning of insulin resistance lacks consensus, several explanations are proposed: direct effect on beta cells of the pancreas, decrease in insulin transporters, insulin receptor malfunction, chronic elevations of fatty acids, and loss of cellular response to insulin signaling.[27,41,42]

A range of evidence suggests that treatment with certain antipsychotic medications is associated with an increased risk of insulin resistance, hyperglycemia, and type 2 diabetes, compared with no treatment or treatment with alternative antipsychotics. Interpretation of the literature has been complicated by reports that patients with major mental disorders such as schizophrenia have an increased prevalence of abnormalities in glucose regulation (e.g., insulin resistance) before the initiation of antipsychotic therapy.

A growing body of evidence supports the key observation that treatments producing the greatest increases in body weight and adiposity are also associated with a consistent pattern of clinically significant adverse effects on insulin resistance and changes in blood glucose and lipid levels. However, there are a growing number of cases of antipsychotic-associated hyperglycemia that involve patients without substantial weight gain, and reports that involve patients who improve when the offending agent is discontinued or who experience deterioration of glycemic control when re-challenged with the drug.[43]

Several summary articles on reports of clozapine and olanzapine-associated hyperglycemia have been published. Cases reported to the FDA's MedWatch Drug Surveillance system were compiled with published cases reported in the literature and/or in national meeting abstracts. Three-hundred eighty-four unique cases of clozapine-associated hyperglycemia and 234 cases of olanzapine-associated hyperglycemia were identified between 1990 and 2001. It is interesting that 78% of clozapine-treated patients and 79% of olanzapine-treated patients had improvements in glycemic control once the putative offending agent was stopped. Additionally, in patients who were rechallenged with the original drug, 75% and 80% of clozapine- and olanzapine-treated patients, respectively, experienced recurrent loss of glycemic control.[43]

Current evidence supports an increase in the risk of diabetes with olanzapine compared to risperidone, although studies are not entirely consistent on this finding. Evidence on the risk of diabetes with quetiapine is more limited, and it appears to be less compared to olanzapine and clozapine.

In the CATIE trial, olanzapine-treated patients showed the greatest increase in glycosylated hemoglobin (A_{1c}) with statistically significant differences between treatment groups in this index.[36]

Since 1994, case reports began to surface in the psychiatric literature suggesting a possible association between the use of SGAs and hyperglycemia. A large number of cases have been reported describing clozapine-associated hyperglycemia.[44-55] Additional reports have surfaced to implicate olanzapine,[56-61] quetiapine,[62-65] and risperidone[46,66,67] as well. With regard to onset, time to onset of newly diagnosed diabetes varied slightly, with 56% and 49% of new cases occurring within the first 3 months for clozapine and olanzapine, respectively.

Although quetiapine has been on the market for a shorter period of time relative to clozapine and olanzapine, a growing number of reports seem to imply that its ability to cause glucoregulatory problems may lie somewhere between that of risperidone and clozapine/olanzapine.[62-65] Ziprasidone and aripiprazole are the newest of the atypical antipsychotics, and data thus far suggest that they cause lower rates of hyperglycemia, although it must be kept in mind that data are limited due to a relative shorter duration of time on the market.

It appears a diagnosis of schizophrenia alone increases the risk of developing diabetes, and this is particularly true for younger patients. A study by Lund et al.[68] compared rates of development of diabetes, hypertension, and hyperlipidemia in patients treated with clozapine versus those treated with typical antipsychotics. This was a retrospective cohort study, which used an analysis of medical claim records to compare 552 clozapine-treated patients with 2,461 typical antipsychotic users. Over the 24-month observation period, a non-significant difference in the occurrence of diabetes was observed between patients receiving clozapine and typical antipsychotics when comparing all ages. When comparing patients 20 to 34 years of age, however, clozapine-treated patients had a significantly greater (2.5-fold) risk of developing diabetes relative to their typically treated counterparts. The authors concluded that clozapine may lead to an earlier onset of diabetes in susceptible patients, but those who will develop diabetes have already done so among the older age groups, so the addition of clozapine does not likely increase the risk.

Several investigators have evaluated the effect of olanzapine on new-onset diabetes. Meyer conducted a retrospective chart review comparing weight, lipid, and glucose changes in risperidone- and olanzapine-treated patients at an Oregon State Hospital in 1999.[69] Patients included in the study had records detailing weight, as well as fasting triglycerides, total cholesterol, and plasma glucose 3 months prior to starting olanzapine or risperidone treatment, and records for these same variables 12 months after initiating the respective agents. Changes in these parameters over the 1-year time period were compared between groups. Olanzapine-treated patients younger than 60 years of age had significant elevations in all parameters relative to risperidone-treated patients, with the exception of weight. When comparing all patients, however, a nonsignificant difference in plasma glucose was apparent. The author in this study noted that increases in plasma glucose did not correlate with increases in weight or with increasing doses of olanzapine.

Another study by Koro et al.[70] used data from the United Kingdom General Practice Database to compare the rates of new-onset diabetes between patients with schizophrenia receiving no antipsychotic agents and those receiving olanzapine, risperidone, or a typical antipsychotic. More than 30 million patient-years were included in the analysis. Investigators included patients who had a diagnosis of schizophrenia, no prior history of diabetes, and at least 3 months of follow-up data after starting an antipsychotic agent. Cases were defined as patients who developed diabetes within 3 months of starting an antipsychotic, and controls were defined as patients who did not. Investigators found that the risk of developing diabetes was significantly elevated for olanzapine-treated patients relative to the typical antipsychotic group. Patients treated with typical antipsychotics had a modest but significantly increased risk of new-onset diabetes relative to the nontreatment group, whereas risperidone-treated patients had nonsignificant increases in risk relative to the nontreatment and typical antipsychotic groups. Unfortunately, this study did not track data on weight change and lacked sufficient power to directly compare olanzapine with risperidone.

More recently, several authors have undertaken large investigations comparing the risk of diabetes associated with multiple agents within one study. Sernyak et al. conducted a nationwide investigation on all patients with schizophrenia treated within the Veterans Health Administration system between June 1999 and September 1999.[40] The researchers compared 22,648 users of atypical antipsychotics with 15,984 users of typical antipsychotics. The study demonstrated that patients were significantly more likely to have diabetes if treated with clozapine, olanzapine, or quetiapine (but not risperidone) compared with patients treated with typical antipsychotics, and these findings were especially true for younger patients. When the atypical antipsychotic group was compared with the typical antipsychotic group, there was a nonsignificant difference of 18.8% versus 18.6%. According to the authors, this was possibly due to the fact that nearly half of the atypical antipsychotic group was being treated with relatively nondiabetogenic risperidone and that the typical antipsychotic group was significantly older. The authors concluded that exposing susceptible younger patients to atypical antipsychotics might hasten the development of the diabetes rather than precipitate it de novo.

A similar study by Gianfrancesco et al. used medical claims data from a health plan database serving 2.5 million people to compare the frequency of newly reported diabetes in psychotic patients receiving high-potency neuroleptics, low-potency neuroleptics, clozapine, olanzapine, and risperidone.[71] The researchers compared each group with a control group consisting of psychotic patients receiving no antipsychotic agents and calculated odds ratios for each agent relative to the control group based on 12 months of exposure. Patients in the clozapine, olanzapine, and low-potency neuroleptic groups had increased odds of developing diabetes. The investigators also found significant correlations between new-onset diabetes and older age, the use of nonantipsychotic agents, and increased olanzapine dose. This study had one major flaw in that the cause of psychosis varied markedly between treatment groups. Specifically, those groups with the lowest odds ratios (i.e., risperidone and high-potency neuroleptics) also had the lowest percentage of patients with schizophrenia; many of these patients had psychotic forms of depression. Because schizophrenia itself is associated with an increased risk of diabetes, it is likely that the inequity between the study groups reduced the odds of diabetes for patients receiving risperidone and high-potency neuroleptics.

Several authors have also used investigational techniques for studying insulin and glucose metabolism to assess the occurrence of antipsychotic-associated hyperglycemia among patients with schizophrenia. The first study of this kind, by Hagg et al., investigated 63 clozapine-treated and 67 typical antipsychotic-treated patients in northern Sweden.[72] To determine rates of impaired glucose tolerance (IGT) and type 2 diabetes in each group, patients underwent two random venous blood draws for plasma glucose. If concentrations exceeded 119 mg/dL, patients were further examined by means of an oral glucose tolerance test (OGTT) according to World Health Organization criteria. Investigators found the prevalence of type 2 diabetes and IGT in the clozapine group to be 12% and 10%, respectively, compared with 6% and 3%, respectively, in the control group. The combined prevalence of type 2 diabetes and IGT in the clozapine group was 22% compared with 10% in the control group ($p = 0.06$). This lack of significance was attributed to a type 2 statistical error, and data were further confounded by the fact that patients in the typical antipsychotic group were significantly older.

Similarly, Newcomer et. al. studied 48 patients with schizophrenia who were taking various antipsychotics (typical n = 17, clozapine n = 9, olanzapine n = 12, risperidone n = 10) and 31 age- and body mass index

(BMI)–matched, healthy controls with a modified OGTT.[73] Patients were excluded from the analysis if they had a previous history of hyperglycemia. The study compared fasting glucose and 15-, 45-, and 75-minute postload glucose and insulin concentrations. The treatment group had significant increases in glucose at all time points relative to healthy controls. Clozapine-treated patients demonstrated significantly increased glucose concentrations (i.e., 1.0–1.5 standard deviations) at all time points relative to the nontreatment group and the typical antipsychotic group. Olanzapine-treated patients demonstrated significantly increased glucose concentrations (i.e., 1.0–1.5 standard deviations) at fasting and 75 minute postload relative to the nontreatment and typical antipsychotic groups. Risperidone-treated patients demonstrated significantly increased glucose concentrations (i.e., 1.0–1.5 standard deviations) at fasting and 45 and 75 minute postload relative to the nontreatment group but not the typical antipsychotic group. No significant differences were found between the typical antipsychotic group and nontreatment groups at any time point.

A large, retrospective pharmacoepidemiological study analyzed prescription claims to determine the relative risk of developing diabetes mellitus among patients treated with a single antipsychotic.[74] Hazard ratios (HRs) for developing diabetes in the combined conventional (HR 3.5, 3.1–3.9 95% CI, $p < 0.0001$), combined atypical (HR 3.1, 2.9–3.4 95% CI, $p < 0.0001$), and individual conventional and atypical antipsychotic treatment cohorts were greater than the general patient population cohort. However, the differences in diabetes rates seen with the individual agents studied were relatively modest, and the risk of diabetes for the combined conventional cohort was not significantly different from that of the combined atypical cohorts (HR 0.97, CI 0.84–1.11; $p = 0.626$). Limitations of this study include a lack of psychiatric diagnostic information (all psychiatric indications were included), and only incident cases of diabetes that resulted in intervention with antidiabetic medications were identified.

Table 4.6 summarizes long-term study results in regards to the incidence of diabetes mellitus among patients on SGAs.

Mechanism of Antipsychotic-Associated Hyperglycemia Antipsychotics may lead to diabetes in susceptible individuals by causing decreased insulin secretion, increased insulin resistance, or a combination of both. Data suggest, however, that insulin resistance is primarily the responsible mechanism. This is supported by the fact that patients treated with clozapine and olanzapine have significant elevations in fasting insulin levels, as well as postload insulin levels during OGTTs compared with healthy controls and patients treated with agents less strongly associated with hyperglycemia.[73] Additionally, authors have demonstrated increased insulin resistance in patients receiving clozapine and olanzapine by homeostatic model assessment, a method used to quantify insulin resistance and beta cell function.[73,75] The mechanism through which antipsychotics lead to insulin resistance is not clear.

Table 4.6 Incidence of diabetes mellitus in comparative long-term observational studies

Study, year indication funder	Interventions	N	Duration (months)	Results
Caro, 2002 Mixed risperidone	Olanzapine Risperidone Mean doses NR	33,946	<3mos to ≥12 mos	Cox Proportional hazard analysis: Olanzapine v risperidone: HR 1.20, 95% CI 1.00 to 1.43, p = 0.05
Fuller, 2003 Mixed risperidone	Olanzapine 10 mg[†] Risperidone 2.8 mg[†]	5,837	NR	Cox regression multivariate analysis: Olanzapine v risperidone: **HR 1.37, 95% CI 1.06 to 1.76**
Ollendorf, 2004 Schizophrenia olanzapine	Olanzapine, olanzapine, quetiapine, risperidone Mean doses NR	2,443	14.5	Cox Proportional hazards HR (95% CI) Olanzapine v risperidone: 1.05 (0.93–1.17) Olanzapine v quetiapine: 1.17 (0.97–1.37) Olanzapine v clozapine: 1.47 (0.97–1.97)
Lee, 2002 Mixed olanzapine	Olanzapine (n = 513) Risperidone (n = 750) Mean doses NR	2,315	12	Logistic Regression Odds Ratio (95% CI) Olanzapine v risperidone: 0.79 (.38–1.61)
Gianfrancesco 2003a Psychosis quetiapine	Olanzapine Quetiapine Risperidone Typical AP Mean doses NR	13,878[§]	8.7 7.1 9.1 12.1	Logistic Regression Odds Ratios v No Treatment* **Olanzapine 1.030, p. = 0.0247** Quetiapine 0.998, p = 0.9593 Risperidone 0.966, p = 0.2848

(Continued)

Table **4.6**	Incidence of diabetes mellitus in comparative long-term observational studies *(Continued)*			
Study, year indication funder	**Interventions**	**N**	**Duration (months)**	**Results**
Gianfrancesco 2002 Psychosis risperidone	Risperidone 2.3 mg[†] Olanzapine 3.6 mg[†] Olanzapine 2.5 mg[†] (risperidone equivalents)	7,933[§]	6.8 6.1 9.4	Logistic Regression Odds Ratios vs No Treatment* **Olanzapine 1.182, p. = 0.0104** **Olanzapine 1.089, p = 0.0006** Risperidone 0.989, p = 0.7650
Gianfrancesco 2003b Mood disorders risperidone	Risperidone 2.1 mg[†] Olanzapine 3.4 mg[†] (risperidone equivalents)	4.387[§]	6.1 6.5	Logistic Regression Odds Ratios vs No Treatment* **Olanzapine 1.129, p. = 0.0001** Risperidone 1.002, p = 0.9582
Koro, 2002 Schizophrenia	Olanzapine Risperidone Typical AP Mean doses NR	3,420	3	Logistic Regression Odds Ratios vs No Treatment* **Olanzapine 5.8; 95%CI; 2.0–16.7** Risperidone 2.2; 95%CI; 0.9–5.2

*LR model using treatment duration as the measurement of exposure.
[§]Includes AAP, Typical AP, and untreated patients.
[†]Doses below midrange.

Reprinted with permission from McDonagh MS, Peterson K, Carson S. Drug Class Review on Atypical Antipsychotic Drugs. Final Report April 2006. Oregon Health & Science University Evidence-based Practice Center. [Online]
http://www.ohsu.edu/drugeffectiveness/reports/documents/AAPs%20Final%20Report%20Update%201.pdf

It has been proposed that antipsychotics may bind insulin receptors, thereby causing decreased affinity of insulin at its receptor site.[76] Additionally, antipsychotics may interfere with the trafficking or kinetics of GLUT4 transporters, leading to either decreased numbers of GLUT4 transporters on the plasma membrane or a decreased half-life of such transporters on the membrane.[77] It is currently unclear which, if any, of these mechanisms is operative. It has also been proposed that atypical antipsychotics lead to diabetes via antagonism of serotonin receptors, particularly the 5-HT1A and 5-HT2 receptors.[76,78] The roles of these receptors in the regulation of glucose metabolism is complex and poorly understood, however, so these theories have not yet been tested. Finally, although increased adiposity has clearly been shown to contribute to insulin resistance and diabetes in the general population, and although many of the atypical antipsychotics lead to substantial increases in adiposity, several studies have failed to show a relationship between weight gain and diabetes associated with atypical antipsychotic use.

Recommendations and Conclusions With Regard to Diabetes Patients with schizophrenia develop diabetes far more frequently than the general population. Additionally, some of the newer antipsychotics, particularly clozapine and olanzapine, appear to be associated with a much higher risk compared with others. Given the profound number of complications associated with diabetes and the tremendous cost to both patients and society that these complications entail, patients prescribed antipsychotics need to be monitored for diabetes more frequently than the general population.

Diagnosing diabetes among patients with schizophrenia is especially difficult because many patients are unaware of the signs and symptoms of the disease and/or lack the ability to communicate this information effectively to their treating physicians. Additionally, many clinicians may dismiss complaints as normal side effects of the antipsychotic medications themselves.

The ADA/APA recommends baseline and annual screening for diabetes or impaired glucose tolerance with fasting glucose and/or an OGTT for all patients started on atypical antipsychotics. The baseline monitoring for the initiation of any antipsychotic medication should include (a) personal and family history of obesity, diabetes, dyslipidemia, hypertension, or cardiovascular disease; (b) weight, height, and BMI; (c) waist circumference; (d) blood pressure; (e) fasting plasma glucose; and (f) fasting lipid profile. Follow-up monitoring should include (a) weight and BMI reassessment at 4 weeks, 8 weeks, and 12 weeks, and quarterly thereafter; (b) waist circumference annually; (c) blood pressure at 12 weeks following initiation and annually thereafter; (d) fasting plasma glucose at 12 weeks following initiation and annually thereafter; and (e) lipid levels 12 weeks following initiation and every 5 years thereafter. The panel also recommends that nutrition and exercise counseling be provided for overweight or obese patients being started on an antipsychotic[28] (Table 4.7),

Table **4.7**	American Diabetes Association/American Psychiatric Association metabolic monitoring recommendations during antipsychotic therapy						
	Baseline	4 weeks	8 weeks	12 weeks	Quarterly	Annually	Every 5 years
Personal/family history	X					X	
Weight (BMI)[a]	X	X	X	X	X		
Waist circumference	X					X	
Blood pressure	X			X		X	
Fasting plasma glucose	X			X		X	
Fasting lipid profile	X			X			X

[a]BMI, body mass index.
From American Diabetes Association, American Psychiatric Association, American Association of Clinical Endocrinologists: Consensus development conference on antipsychotic drugs and obesity and diabetes. *Diabetes Care* 2004;27(2):596–601, with permission.

Additionally, glucose screening should occur before and after antipsychotic regimens are changed. If and when abnormalities are detected during these monitoring practices, patients should be referred quickly to primary care physicians for initiation of treatment and monitoring for complications.

Effects on Lipids Dyslipidemia is a condition in which lipid levels are not normal, and it is associated with atypical antipsychotic drug use. Further, diabetic dyslipidemia is a chief feature of CVD, which in turn is a major factor in premature death. Specifically, dyslipidemia has a characteristic triad of lipid alterations consisting of one or more of the following: increased levels of LDL cholesterol, lowered levels of HDL cholesterol, and elevated triglycerides all working to speed an atherosclerotic process. Dyslipidemia risk factors can be reduced, yet medical supervision in individuals with schizophrenia is less intense than for people in the general population.

Results from numerous studies suggest that triglyceride levels do increase significantly in patients being treated with either clozapine or olanzapine. A scarcity of case reports revolving around risperidone and quetiapine suggests that changes in triglycerides occur less frequently with these agents. Although the mechanism behind elevations in triglycerides is largely unknown, it may occur in relation to weight gain.

In the CATIE trial, olanzapine-treated patients showed the greatest increases in total cholesterol (mean increase 9.7 mg/dL, standard deviation [SD] = 2.1) and triglycerides (mean increase 42.9 mg/dL, SD = 8.4), with statistically significant differences between treatment groups in both of these indices.[36]

A study by Ghaeli and Dufresne found increased serum triglyceride levels after initiation of treatment with clozapine without a significant change in serum cholesterol.[79] In a 5-year naturalistic study of the effects of clozapine among 82 patients, there was a significant and persistent increase in serum triglyceride levels, and there was a nonsignificant increase on serum cholesterol levels. [80]

A retrospective review of the charts of 590 patients compared several SGAs (clozapine, risperidone, olanzapine, and quetiapine) with each other and with the typical agents (fluphenazine and haloperidol) in regard to their propensity to affect lipid parameters.[81] Of the patients reviewed, 215 subjects had adequate laboratory data for inclusion. The authors found that patients receiving clozapine and olanzapine showed significant increases in triglyceride levels compared with the other groups (triglyceride levels increased more than 30% for clozapine and olanzapine compared with 19% for risperidone; patients on haloperidol and fluphenazine developed decreases in triglyceride levels). Patients taking olanzapine, risperidone, and quetiapine also showed significant decreases in LDL; in addition, patients taking clozapine and olanzapine also experienced decreases in HDL.

Tables 4.8, 4.9, and 4.10 summarize a number of metabolic adverse events associated with the SGAs.

Mood Stabilizers

Lithium has long been known to have been associated with weight gain. More recently, there is a growing database on anticonvulsants, especially valproic acid or divalproex sodium in regards to its effect on weight gain.

Lithium: Extensive clinical experience and well-controlled studies show that lithium is effective in preventing both manic and depressive episodes of bipolar disorder. Lithium has antidepressant effects and is sometimes used to augment other antidepressants in refractory patients. Lithium may be less effective for severe mania with psychotic features, mixed episodes, rapid/continuous cycling, and inorganic-induced mood states. Lithium carbonate has also been used in the treatment of schizophrenia, schizoaffective disorder, impulse control disorders, aggression, self-injurious behavior, pervasive developmental disorders, mental retardation, alcoholism, substance abuse, bulimia nervosa, premenstrual syndrome, and steroid-induced mania.

There is no unified theory for its mode of action. Lithium affects the synthesis, storage, release, and reuptake of central monoamine neurotransmitters,

Table 4.8 Selected adverse outcomes from the 2005 CATIE trial

Change from baseline	Olanzapine (n = 336)	Quetiapine (n = 337)	Risperidone (n = 341)	Perphenazine (n = 261)	Ziprasidone (n = 185)	P value
Weight gain more than 7% (%)	92/307 (30)	49/305 (16)	42/300 (14)	29/243 (12)	12/161 (7)	<0.001
Mean weight change (lb)	9.4 ± 0.9	1.1 ± 0.9	0.8 ± 0.9	−2.0 ± 1.1	−1.6 ± 1.1	<0.001
Weight change (lb/month of treatment)	2.0 ± 0.3	0.5 ± 0.2	0.4 ± 0.3	−0.2 ± 0.2	−0.3 ± 0.3	<0.001
$A1_C$ (%) exposure-adjusted mean	0.40 ± 0.07	0.04 ± 0.08	0.07 ± 0.08	0.09 ± 0.09	0.11 ± 0.09	0.01
Cholesterol (mg/dL)	9.7 ± 2.1	5.3 ± 2.1	−2.1 ± 1.9	0.5 ± 2.3	−9.2 ± 5.2	<0.001
Triglycerides (mg/dL)	42.9 ± 8.4	19.2 ± 10.6	−2.6 ± 6.3	8.3 ± 11.5	−18.1 ± 9.4	<0.001
Prolactin (ng/dL) exposure-adjusted mean	−8.1 ± 1.4	−10.6 ± 1.4	13.8 ± 1.4	−1.2 ± 1.6	−5.6 ± 1.9	<0.001
Prolonged QT interval (% patients)	0	3	3	1	1	0.03

Table 4.9 Selected side effects of antipsychotics

Medication	Extra-pyramidal side effects/ tardrve dyskinesia	Prolactin elevation	Weight gain	Glucose abnormalities	Lipid abnormalities	QTc prolongation	Sedation	Hypotension	Anti-cholinergic side effects
Thioridazine	+	++	+	+?	+?	+++	++	++	++
Perphenazine	++	++	+	+?	+?	0	+	+	0
Haloperidol	+++	+++	+	0	0	0	++	0	0
Clozapine[a]	0[b]	0	+++	+++	+++	0	+++	+++	+++
Risperidone	+	+++	++	++	++	+	+	+	0
Olanzapine	0[b]	0	+++	+++	+++	0	+	+	++
Quetiapine[c]	0[b]	0	++	++	++	0	++	++	0
Ziprasidone	0[b]	+	0	0	0	++	0	0	0
Aripiprazole[d]	0[b]	0	0	0	0	0	+	0	0

0 = No risk or rarely causes side effects at therapeutic dose. + = Mild or occasionally causes side effects at therapeutic dose. +++ = Frequently causes side effects at therapeutic dose. ++ = Sometimes causes side effects at therapeutic dose. ? = Data too limited to rate with confidence.

[a]Also causes agranulocytosis, seizures, and myocarditis.

[b]Possible exception of akathisia.

[c]Also carries warning about potential development of cataracts.

[d]Also causes nausea and headache.

Reprinted with permission from American Psychiatric Association. Practice guidelines for the treatment of patients with schizophrenia, Quick Reference Guide. [Online] http://www.psych.org/psych_pract/treatg/quick_ref_guide/Schizophrenia_QRG.pdf

Table **4.10**	Metabolic abnormalities associated with atypical antipsychotics		
Drug	Weight gain	Risk for diabetes	Worsening lipid profile
Clozapine	+++	+	+
Olanzapine	+++	+	+
Risperidone	++	D	D
Quetiapine	++	D	D
Aripiprazole*	+/−	−	−
Ziprasidone*	+/−	−	−

+ = increase effect; = no effect; D = discrepant results. * Newer drugs with limited long-term data.
Reprinted with permission from American Diabetes Association, American Psychiatric Association, American Association of Clinical Endocrinologists: Consensus development conference on antipsychotic drugs and obesity and diabetes. *Diabetes Care* 2004;27(2):596–601.

including NE, 5-HT, dopamine, acetylcholine, and gamma-aminobutyric acid (GABA). Neuropharmacologic effects of lithium include blockade of dopamine-receptor supersensitivity, decreases of beta-adrenoreceptor stimulation of adenylate cyclase, and increases of 5-HT, acetylcholine, and GABA function. Gastrointestinal disturbances (nausea, diarrhea, anorexia, abdominal pain, and bloating) occur in 10% to 30% of patients and are generally mild and transient. Muscle weakness and lethargy, usually transient, are reported in about 30% of patients. Polydipsia with polyuria and nocturia occur in up to 7% of patients (innocuous and diminish with time). Many patients respond to polydipsia with weight gain, probably because of increased consumption of high-calorie fluids or fluid retention. As many as 40% of patients may complain of headache, memory impairment, mental confusion, a decreased ability to concentrate, and impaired fine motor performance. A fine hand tremor may be observed in up to 50% of patients during the first week of lithium therapy, and this usually decreases in intensity with time. Lithium reduces the kidney's ability to concentrate urine and in some patients produces a nephrogenic diabetes insipidus manifested as polyuria. Lithium also blocks thyroid hormone synthesis. Up to 30% of patients on maintenance lithium therapy develop transiently elevated thyroid-stimulating hormone concentrations, and 5% to 15% of patients develop a goiter and/or hypothyroidism.

Effects on Weight Lithium causes weight gain in 30% to 65% of patients.[82–84] Documented mechanisms include insulin-like actions on carbohydrate and fat metabolism, polydipsia, and sodium retention.[85] The etiology of weight gain with lithium is not clear.

Six studies have reported the prevalence of lithium-induced weight gain.[85] The duration of lithium treatment ranged from 6 months to 17 years. Four studies reported weight gain of more than 4.5 kg in 11 to 64% of patients. Two studies reported 20% of patients gained more than 10 kg. This compares with a weight gain of more than 4.5 kg in 8% of affective disorder patients treated with placebo. Overall, the range of weight gained was 3 to 28 kg, with an average of 8.5 kg. Factors associated with weight gain were increased thirst, a previous history of weight problems, and edema, although the latter was not a consistent finding.[85] It is of interest that lithium responders may gain more weight than nonresponders.

Effects on Glucose Lithium may have an insulin-like effect to decrease blood glucose and inhibit adenyl cyclase to decrease lipolysis. Under certain experimental conditions, and particularly in animal experiments, lithium can exhibit insulin-like effects. However, the insulin-induced release of glucose may also be inhibited. A number of researchers have conducted GTTs on patients receiving long-term lithium therapy. These tests have yielded contradictory results. The early reports of slight lithium-induced increases in plasma glucose in humans have not been confirmed by more recent studies.[86,87] In an extensive review of the literature, Lazarus could not confirm a clinically relevant diabetogenic effect in humans.[88]

Carbamazepine: Studies show that the anticonvulsant carbamazepine has acute antimanic, antidepressant, and prophylactic effects comparable with lithium in bipolar disorder. Carbamazepine has been used off-label for mania since the late 1970s, but the FDA approved an extended-release form (Equetro) for bipolar disorder in 2006. Structurally related to TCAs, carbamazepine blocks the reuptake of NE, decreases the release of NE, increases acetylcholine in the stratum, decreases dopamine and GABA turnover, and decreases the activity of adenylate cyclase.

Central nervous system toxicity can occur in up to 60% of patients receiving carbamazepine. Neurologic side effects include drowsiness, dizziness, fatigue, clumsiness, ataxia, vertigo, blurred vision, diplopia, nystagmus, dysarthria, confusion, and headache. Gastrointestinal side effects occur in up to 15% of patients and include nausea, vomiting, abdominal pain, diarrhea, constipation, and anorexia. These effects can be minimized by administering the drug with food or reducing the daily dose. Hypersensitivity develops in 8% to 15% of patients.

Effects on Weight In recent studies of bipolar disorder by the FDA with extended-release carbamazepine, the mean weight gain was 1.0 kg versus 0.1 kg with placebo in a 3-week trial.[89] The mean weight gain in a 6-month extension study was a low 0.7% (equivalent to 0.5 kg in a 70-kg man), suggesting that weight gain in bipolar patients is minimal during long-term treatment with extended-release carbamazepine.[90] Studies suggest a low rate of weight gain with carbamazepine ranging from 2.5% to 14% in patients with epilepsy.[91]

Valproic Acid (Valproate) and Divalproex Sodium: A smaller number of controlled trials and a larger number of open-label studies support the efficacy of valproic acids or divalproex sodium in bipolar disorder. Both carbamazepine and valproate are effective in a large number of lithium-resistant patients with bipolar disorder. The exact mechanism of action of valproate is not known but may be related to the inhibition of GABA metabolism, stimulation of GABA synthesis and release, and augmentation of the postsynaptic inhibitory effect of GABA.

Compared with other anticonvulsants, valproate has a lower incidence of adverse events and is generally well-tolerated. The most frequent adverse effects reported with valproic acid are gastrointestinal complaints (nausea, vomiting, epigastric cramping, dyspepsia, indigestion, and anorexia) and sedation.

Effects on Weight Valproate frequently may cause significant weight gain, an effect that may be mediated in part by the tendency to increase insulin and thereby stimulate appetite.[92] Several clinical studies have described a significant weight gain and increase in serum leptin levels in the course of antiepileptic treatment with valproic acid.[93] A review of weight gain with valproate shows that up to 71% of patients with epilepsy gained weight with valproate.[91] Polycystic ovarian syndrome has been associated with valproate in some but not all studies, and weight gain along with androgen excess has been posited as a mechanism for this disorder.[94] In an analysis of food intake compared with energy expenditure of patients treated with valproate, those with weight gain manifested a lower metabolic rate rather than increased caloric intake.[95]

Effects on Glucose Valproate, a fatty acid derivative, competes with free fatty acids for albumin binding and acts as a GABA-ergic agonist, mechanisms that are known to be involved in pancreatic beta-cell regulation and insulin secretion.[93]

Lamotrigine: Lamotrigine is an anticonvulsant that appears to be an effective mood stabilizer for maintenance treatment of bipolar disorder and may be particularly advantageous in treating depressed mood.[96] Lamotrigine regulates the release of glutamate and aspartate, which are excitatory neurotransmitters.

Adverse events most frequently reported with lamotrigine include diplopia, drowsiness, ataxia, and headache. It may cause several types of rash, which usually appear in the first 3 to 4 weeks of therapy. The rash is typically generalized, erythematous, and morbilliform, and is generally mild to moderate in severity. However, the Stevens-Johnson reaction has also been reported.

Effects on Weight Like carbamazepine, lamotrigine causes little if any weight gain. In a survey of 32 studies including 463 patients, the mean change in body weight was 0.5 ($\pm$ 5) kg.[97]

Table **4.11** Drugs that can increase blood glucose levels	
Name of drug/class	**Clinical significance**
Asparaginase	+ +
Atypical antipsychotic agents	+ + +
Beta agonists	+ +
Beta adrenergic blockers	+ +
Calcitonin	+
Calcium antagonists	+
Carbamazepine	+
Cimetidine	+
Corticosteroids	+ + +
Cyclosporine	+ +
Diazoxide	+ + +
Didanosine	+
Diuretics	+ + +
Encainide	+
Imipramine	+
Isoniazid	+
Lithium	+
Marijuana	+ +
Megestrol acetate	+
Nicotinic acid	+ +
Oral contraceptives	+ +
Pentamidine	+ + +
Phenothiazines	+
Phenytoin	+ +
Pravastatin	+
Protease inhibitors	+ + +
Rifampin	+
Sympathomimetics	+ +
Tacrolimus	+ +
Thyroid hormones	+

From Carlisle BA, Kroon LA, Koda-Kimble MA. Diabetes mellitus. In: Koda-Kimble MA et al., eds. *Applied therapeutics: the clinical use of drugs.* Philadelphia, PA: Lippincott, Williams, & Wilkins; 2005:50.1–50.86, with permission.

Topiramate: Topiramate, which is indicated for epilepsy, is not approved for bipolar disorder due to failed clinical trials. However, it has been noted to induce weight loss and is sometimes used (off-label) to counteract the weight gain induced by other agents.[98–100]

Anxiolytics

Benzodiazepines: Benzodiazepines work by enhancing the inhibitory effects of GABA. These agents are used to treat a wide variety of medical and psychiatric conditions including muscle spasms, seizures, anxiety disorders, agitation, and insomnia, and for the induction of conscious sedation.

Sedation is the most common side effect of the benzodiazepines. Benzodiazepines are also associated with cognitive impairment and potential for tolerance, abuse, and dependence.[101]

Buspirone: Buspirone is a nonbenzodiazepine anxiolytic that works as a partial agonist of the $5HT_{1A}$ receptor. It is indicated in the treatment of generalized anxiety disorder and considered to be relatively free of the potential for abuse and dependence.[101]

Effects on Weight and Glucose In clinical trials, benzodiazepines and buspirone have not been associated with weight gain or alterations in glucose homeostasis.

Other Drugs Associated With Glucose Abnormalities

Many drugs may influence glucose insulin homeostasis. Commonly prescribed drugs that may have adverse effects on carbohydrate metabolism, especially in patients with diabetes mellitus or those at risk of developing glucose intolerance, include diuretics, beta-blockers, sympathomimetics, corticosteroids, and sex hormones (Table 4.11).

References

1. Dixon L, Weiden P, Delahanty J, et al. Prevalence and correlates of diabetes in national schizophrenia samples. *Schizophr Bull.* 2000;26:903–912.
2. Deshmukh R, Franco K. Managing weight gain as a side effect of antidepressant therapy. *Cleve Clin J Med.* 2003;70(7):614–623. http://www.ccjm.org/pdffiles/Deshmuhk703.pdf. Accessed September 10, 2007.
3. Fava M. Weight gain and antidepressants. *J Clin Psychiatry.* 2000;61 (suppl 1): 37–41.
4. Tesar G. Depression and other mood disorders. Cleveland Clinic 2002. http://www.clevelandclinicmeded.com/medicalpubs/diseasemanagement/psychiatry/depression/depression.htm. Accessed September 10, 2007.
5. MacHale S. Managing depression in physical illness. *Adv Psychiatr Treat.* 2002;8:297–306.

6. Feighner JP. Cardiovascular safety in depressed patients: focus on venlafaxine. *J Clin Psychiatry.* 1995;56(12):574–579.
7. Silverstone PH, Ravindran A. Once-daily venlafaxine extended release compared with fluoxetine in outpatients with depression and anxiety. Venlafaxine XR 360 Study Group. *J Clin Psychiatry.* 1999;60(1):22–28.
8. Wells BG, Mandos LA, Hays PE. Depressive disorders. In: DiPiro J, ed. *Pharmacotherapy: a pathophysiologic approach.* 3rd ed. Stamford, CT: Appleton & Lange, 1997:1395–1417.
9. FDA MedWatch [Dear Healthcare Provider Letter]. June 2002. http://www.fda. gov/medwatch/SAFETY/2002/serzone_deardoc.PDF. Accessed September 10, 2007.
10. Fieger AD, Bielski RJ, Bikoff J, et al. Double-blind, placebo-substitution study of nefazodone in the prevention of relapse during continuation of treatment of outpatients with major depression. *Int Clin Psychopharmacol.* 1999;14:19–28.
11. Sussman N, Ginsberg DL, Bikoff J. Effects of nefazodone on body weight: a pooled analysis of SSRI and imipramine controlled trials. *J Clin Psychiatry.* 2001;62:256–260.
12. Croft H, Houser TL, Jamerson BD, et al. Effect on body-weight of bupropion sustained release in patients with major depression treated for 52 weeks. *Clin Ther.* 2002;24(4):662–672.
13. Schatzberg AF, Kremer C, Rodrigues HE, et al. Double-blind, randomized comparison of mirtazapine and paroxetine in elderly depressed patients. *Am J Geriatr Psychiatry.* 2002;10(5):541–550.
14. Benkert O, Szegedi A, Kohnen R. Mirtazapine compared with paroxetine in major depression. *J Clin Psychiatry.* 2000;61(9):656–663.
15. Montgomery SA, Reimitz PE, Zivkov M. Mirtazapine versus amitriptyline in the long-term treatment of depression. *Int Clin Psychopharmacol.* 1998;13:63–73.
16. Guelfi JD, Ansseau M, Timmerman L, et al. Mirtazapine vs. venlafaxine in hospitalized severely depressed patients with melancholic features. Mirtazapine-Venlafaxine Study Group. *J Clin Psychopharmacol.* 2001;21:425–431.
17. Remeron® prescribing information. Organon, Inc. Remeron package insert. West Orange, NJ: April 1996.
18. Nicholas LM, Ford AL, Esposito SM, et al. The effects of mirtazapine on plasma lipid profiles in healthy subjects. *J Clin Psychiatry.* 2003;64:883–889.
19. Cantu TG, Korek JS. Monoamine oxidase inhibitors and weight gain. *Drug Intell Clin Pharm.* 1988;22:755–779.
20. EMSAM (selegiline transdermal system) Prescribing Information. Tampa, FL: Somerset Pharmaceuticals, Inc; 2006.
21. Pandit MK, Burke J, Gustafson AB, et al. Drug-induced disorders of glucose tolerance. *Ann Intern Med.* 1993;118(7):529–539.
22. American Psychiatric Association. Practice guidelines for the treatment of patients with major depressive disorder. *Am J Psychiatry.* 2000;suppl 4:1–45.
23. Gartlehner G, Hansen RA, Kahwati L, et al. Drug class review on second generation antidepressants. Final Report September 2006. Oregon Health & Science University. Evidence-based Practice Center. http://www.ohsu.edu/drugeffectiveness/reports/documents/SG%20Antidepressants%20Final%20Report%20u3.pdf. Accessed September 10, 2007.

24. Fava M, Rosenbaum JF, Hoog SL, et al. Fluoxetine versus sertraline and paroxetine in major depression: changes in weight with long-term treatment. *J Clin Psychiatry.* 2000;61(11):863–867.

25. Maina G, Albert U, Salvi V, et al. Weight gain during long-term treatment of obsessive-compulsive disorder: a prospective comparison between serotonin reuptake inhibitors. *J Clin Psychiatry.* 2004;65(10):1365–1371.

26. Bazire S. *Psychotropic drug directory: the professionals' pocket handbook and aide memoire.* Lancaster: Quay Publishing Ltd., 2001.

27. Petty R. *Diabetes in schizophrenia.* Tucker, GA: The Promedica Research Center, 2003.

28. American Diabetes Association, American Psychiatric Association, American Association of Clinical Endocrinologists: Consensus development conference on antipsychotic drugs and obesity and diabetes. *Diabetes Care.* 2004;27(2):596–601.

29. World Health Organization. Definition, diagnosis and classification of diabetes mellitus and its complications. Geneva: 1999. http://whqlibdoc.who.int/hq/1999/WHO_NCD_NCS_99.2.pdf. Accessed September 10, 2007.

30. Kawachi I. Health consequences of weight gain. *Ther Adv Psychoses.* 1999;7:1–3.

31. Newcomer JW. Second-generation (atypical) antipsychotics and metabolic effects: a comprehensive literature review. *CNS Drugs.* 2005;19(Suppl 1):1–93.

32. Allison DB, Mentore JL, Heo M, et al. Antipsychotic-induced weight-gain: a comprehensive research synthesis. *Am J Psychiatry.* 1999;156:1686–1696.

33. Leucht S, Wagenpfeil S, Hamann J, et al. Amisulpride is an "atypical" antipsychotic associated with low weight gain. *Psychopharmacology.* 2004;173:112–115.

34. Newcomer JW, Haupt DW. The metabolic effects of antipsychotic medications. *Can J Psychiatry.* 2006;51(8):480–491.

35. Nemeroff CB. Dosing the antipsychotic olanzapine. *J Clin Psychiatry.* 1997;58(Suppl 10):45–49.

36. Lieberman JA, Stroup TS, McEvoy JP, et al., for the Clinical Antipsychotic Trials of Intervention Effectiveness (CATIE) Investigators. Effectiveness of antipsychotic drugs in patients with chronic schizophrenia. *N Engl J Med.* 2005; 353:1209–1223.

37. McDonagh MS, Peterson K, Carson S. Drug class review on atypical antipsychotic drugs. Final Report April 2006. Oregon Health & Science University Evidence-based Practice Center. http://www.ohsu.edu/drugeffectiveness/reports/documents/AAPs%20Final%20Report%20Update%201.pdf. Accessed on: September 10, 2007.

38. McQuade RD, Stock E, Marcus R, et al. A comparison of weight change during treatment with olanzapine or aripiprazole: results from a randomized, double-blind study. *J Clin Psychiatry.* 2004;65 Suppl 18:47–56.

39. Basson BR, Kinon BJ, Taylor CC, et al. Factors influencing acute weight change in patients with schizophrenia treated with olanzapine, haloperidol, or risperidone. *J Clin Psychiatry.* 2001;62:231–238.

40. Sernyak MJ, Leslie DL, Alarcon RD, et al. Association of diabetes mellitus with use of atypical neuroleptics in the treatment of schizophrenia. *Am Jf Psychiatry.* 2002;159(4):561–566.

41. Birkenaes AB, Andreassen OA. The metabolic side effects of antipsychotic medications. *Psychiatry Rev Ser.* 2004;4:4–7.

42. Carmena R. Type 2 diabetes, dyslipidemia, and vascular risk: rationale and evidence for correcting the lipid imbalance. *Am Heart J.* 2005;150(5):859–870.

43. Clark C, Burge MR. Diabetes mellitus associated with atypical antipsychotic medications. *Diabetes Technol Ther.* 2003;5(4):669–683.
44. Maule S, Giannella R, Lanzio M, et al. Diabetic ketoacidosis with clozapine treatment. *Diabetes Nutr Metab.* 1999;12(2):187–188.
45. Colli A, Cocciolo M, Francobandiera F, et al. Diabetic ketoacidosis associated with clozapine treatment. *Diabetes Care.* 1999;22(1):176–177.
46. Mohan D, Gordon H, Hindley N, et al. Schizophrenia and diabetes mellitus. *Br J Psychiatry.* 1999;174:180–181.
47. Smith H, Kenney-Herbert J, Knowles L. Clozapine-induced diabetic ketoacidosis. *Aust N Z J Psychiatry.* 1999;33(1):120–121.
48. Ai D, Roper TA, Riley JA. Diabetic ketoacidosis and clozapine. *Postgrad Med J.* 1998;74(874):493–494.
49. Wirshing DA, Spellberg BJ, Erhart SM, et al. Novel antipsychotics and new onset diabetes. *Biol Psychiatry.* 1998;44(8):778–783.
50. Markowitz JS, Gill HS, Devane CL, et al. Fluoroquinolone inhibition of clozapine metabolism. *Am J Psychiatry.* 1997;154(6):881.
51. Popli AP, Konicki PE, Jurjus GJ, et al. Clozapine and associated diabetes mellitus. *J Clin Psychiatry.* 1997;58(3):108–111.
52. Peterson GA, Byrd SL. Diabetic ketoacidosis from clozapine and lithium cotreatment. *Am J Psychiatry.* 1996;153(5):737–738.
53. Kostakoglu AE, Yazici KM, Erbas T, et al. Ketoacidosis as a side-effect of clozapine: a case report. *Acta Psychiatr Scand.* 1996;93(3):217–218.
54. Koval MS, Rames LJ, Christie S. Diabetic ketoacidosis associated with clozapine treatment. *Am J Psychiatry.* 1994;151(10):1520–1521.
55. Kamran A, Doraiswamy PM, Jane JL, et al. Severe hyperglycemia associated with high doses of clozapine. *Am J Psychiatry.* 1994;151(9):1395.
56. Bettinger TL, Mendelson SC, Dorson PG, et al. Olanzapine-induced glucose dysregulation. *Ann Pharmacother.* 2000;34(7–8):865–867.
57. Goldstein LE, Sporn J, Brown S, et al. New-onset diabetes mellitus and diabetic ketoacidosis associated with olanzapine treatment. *Psychosomatics.* 1999;40(5): 438–443.
58. Gatta B, Rigalleau V, Gin H. Diabetic ketoacidosis with olanzapine treatment. *Diabetes Care.* 1999;22(6):1002–1003.
59. Ober SK, Hudak R, Rusterholtz A. Hyperglycemia and olanzapine. *Am J Psychiatry.* 1999;156(6):970.
60. Fertig MK, Brooks VG, Shelton PS, et al. Hyperglycemia associated with olanzapine. *J Clin Psychiatry.* 1998;59(12):687–689.
61. Melkersson KI, Hulting AL, Brismar KE. Elevated levels of insulin, leptin, and blood lipids in olanzapine-treated patients with schizophrenia or related psychoses. *J Clin Psychiatry* 2000;61(10):742–749.
62. Wilson DR, D'Souza L, Sarkar N, et al. New-onset diabetes and ketoacidosis with atypical antipsychotics. *Schizophr Res.* 2003;59(1):1–6.
63. Procyshyn RM, Pande S, Tse G. New-onset diabetes mellitus associated with quetiapine. *Can J Psychiatry.* 2000;45:668–669.
64. Sobel M, Jaggers ED, Franz MA. New-onset diabetes mellitus associated with quetiapine [letter]. *J Clin Psychiatry.* 1999;60:556–557.
65. Domon SE, Cargile CS. Quetiapine-associated hyperglycemia and hypertriglyceridemia. *J Am Acad Child Adolesc Psychiatry.* 2003;41:495–496.

66. Croakin PE, Jacobs KM, Bain BK. Diabetic ketoacidosis associated with risperidone treatment? *Psychosomatics.* 2000;41:369–370.

67. Wirshing DA, Erhart SM, Pierre JM, et al. Nonextrapyramidal side effects of novel antipsychotics. *Curr Opin Psychiatry.* 2000;13:45–50.

68. Lund BC, Perry PJ, Brooks JM, et al. Clozapine use in patients with schizophrenia and the risk of diabetes, hyperlipidemia, and hypertension. *Arch Gen Psychiatry.* 2001;58:1172–1176.

69. Meyer JM. A retrospective comparison of weight, lipid, and glucose changes between risperidone- and olanzapine-treated inpatients: metabolic outcomes after 1 year. *J Clin Psychiatry.* 2002;63(5):425–433.

70. Koro CE, Fedder DO, L'Italien GJ, et al. Assessment of independent effects of olanzapine and risperidone on the risk of diabetes among patients with schizophrenia: population based nested case control. *BMJ.* 2002;325:243–245.

71. Gianfrancesco FD, Grogg AL, Mahmond RA, et al. Differential effects of risperidone, olanzapine, clozapine and conventional antipsychotics on type 2 diabetes: findings from a large health plan database. *J Clin Psychiatry.* 2002;63:920–930.

72. Hagg S, Joelsson L, Mjorndal T, et al. Prevalence of diabetes and impaired glucose tolerance in patients treated with clozapine compared to patients treated with conventional depot neuroleptic medications. *J Clin Psychiatry.* 1998;59: 294–299.

73. Newcomer JW, Haupt DW, Fucetola R, et al. Abnormalities in glucose regulation during antipsychotics treatment of schizophrenia. *Arch Gen Psychiatry.* 2002;59: 337–345.

74. Buse JB, Cavazzoni P, Hornbuckel K, et al. A retrospective cohort study of diabetes mellitus and antipsychotic treatment in the United States. *J Clin Epidemiol.* 2003;56:164–170.

75. Fryburg D, O'Sullivan R, Siu C, et al. Insulin resistance in olanzapine- and ziprasidone-treated patients: interim results of a double-blind controlled 6-week trial. Presented at the 39th annual meeting of the American College of Neuropsychopharmacology, Dec 10–14, 2000; San Juan, Puerto Rico.

76. Dwyer DS, Bradley RJ, Kablinger AS, et al. Glucose metabolism in relation to schizophrenia and antipsychotic drug treatment. *Ann Clin Psychiatry.* 2001;13: 103–113.

77. Goldstein L, Henderson D. Atypical antipsychotic agents and diabetes mellitus. *Prim Psychiatry.* 2000;7:65–68.

78. Haupt DW, Newcomer JW. Hyperglycemia and antipsychotic medication. *J Clin Psychiatry.* 2001;62(Suppl 27):15–26.

79. Ghaeli P, Dufresne RL. Serum triglyceride level in patients treated with clozapine. *Am J Health Syst Pharm.* 1996;53:2079–2081.

80. Henderson DC, Cagliero E, Gray C. Clozapine, diabetes mellitus, weight gain, and lipid abnormalities: a five-year naturalistic study. *Am J Psychiatry.* 2000;157: 975–981.

81. Wirshing DA, Boyd JA, Meng LR, et al. The effects of novel antipsychotic medications on weight gain, glucose, and lipid levels. *J Clin Psychiatry.* 2002;63: 856–865.

82. Aronne LJ, Segal KR. Weight gain in the treatment of mood disorders. *J Clin Psychiatry.* 2003;64(suppl 8):22–29.

83. Baptista T, Teneud L, Contreras Q, et al. Lithium and body weight gain. *Pharmacopsychiatry.* 1995;28:35–44.

Chapter 4 • Psychotropic Medications and Metabolic Disorders **83**

---

104. Goodnick PJ, Breakstone K, Kumar A, et al. Nefazodone in diabetic neuropathy: response and biology [letter to the editor]. *Psychosom Med.* 2000;62(4):599–600.
105. Isotani H, Kameoka K. Hypoglycemia associated with maprotiline in a patient with type 1 diabetes. *Diabetes Care.* 1999; 22(5):862–863.
106. Kennedy SH, Evans KR, Kruger S, et al. Changes in regional brain glucose metabolism measured with positron emission tomography after paroxetine treatment of major depression. *Am J Psychiatry.* 2001;158(6):899–905.
107. Pollak PT, Mukherjee SD, Fraser AD. Sertraline-induced hypoglycemia. *Ann Pharmacother.* 2001; 35(11):1371–1374.
108. Rowland MJ, Bransome ED, Hendry LB. Hypoglycemia caused by selegiline, an antiparkinsonian drug: can such side effects be predicted? *J Clin Pharmacol.* 1994;34:80–85.
109. Warlock JK, Biggs F. Nefazodone-induced hypoglycemia in a diabetic patient with major depression [letter to the editor]. *Am J Psychiatry.* 1997;154(2):288–289.
110. Goodnick PJ. Use of antidepressants in treatment of comorbid diabetes mellitus and depression as well as in diabetic neuropathy. *Ann Clin Psychiatry.* 2001; 13(1):31–41.
111. McIntyre RS, Soczynska JK, et al. The effect of antidepressants on glucose homeostasis and insulin sensitivity: synthesis and mechanisms. *Expert Opin Drug Safety.* 2006;5(1):157–168.
112. Smith GS, Ma Y, Dhawan V, et al. Serotonin modulation of cerebral glucose metabolism measured with positron emission tomography (PET) in human subjects. *Synapse.* 2002;45(2):105–112.
113. Grundy SM. Metabolic syndrome scientific statement by the American Heart Association and the National Heart, Lung, and Blood Institute. *Arterioscl Thromb Vasc Biol.* 2005;24:2243–2244.
114. American Psychiatric Association. Practice guidelines for the treatment of patients with schizophrenia, Quick Reference Guide. http://www.psych.org/psych_pract/treatg/quick_ref_guide/Schizophrenia_QRG.pdf. Accessed September 7, 2007.

CHAPTER 5

Interventions

Jennifer A. Rosen, Arlene E. Johns,
Shahla S. Cano, and Eda Vesterman

Scope of the Problem

It is estimated that 66% of U.S. adults are either overweight or obese.[1] Furthermore, studies indicate that obesity is more prevalent among Americans with serious mental illnesses versus those without mental illnesses.[2] Given the prior discussions of the prevelance of diabetes amongst the mentally ill, it is clear that patients with mental illness possess multiple risk factors for coronary artery disease. This is further compounded by the fact that many medications used to treat mental illnesses contribute to weight gain and the development of diabetes and hypertriglyceridemia.

Much has been said about the cardiovascular problems associated with obesity. However, there may be yet more problems associated with obesity in the mentally ill. Interestingly, distress with regard to weight gain has been shown to be the primary mediator of antipsychotic nonadherence in patients with schizophrenia. Obese individuals with schizophrenia have been reported to be more than twice as likely to report missing their medication, compared with patients with a normal body mass index (BMI).[3]

Of the many factors that increase a patient's risk of diabetes, body weight and diet are two factors than can be controlled. Although managing diet and behavior in the mentally ill population can be challenging, there have been numerous studies that demonstrate effective ways to manage weight gain in the mentally ill.[4] The basic principles of weight management or weight loss are similar to those well-established tenets for the management of weight gain in the general population.[4] For example, improving food choices, restricting portion size, and increasing physical activity have been demonstrated to be necessary components of successful weight loss.[5]

Definition of Overweight and Obesity: The definitions of "overweight" and "obesity" relate to BMI. BMI is calculated using a patient's weight and height, as follows:

$$BMI = Weight\ (kg)/Height^2\ (meters)$$
or
$$Weight\ (lb) \times 703/Height^2\ (inches)$$

Table 5.1 outlines the World Health Organization (WHO) classifications of obesity according to BMI. BMI generally correlates with body fatness, except in cases of elite athletes and body builders. There are also recognized differences according to race, age, and gender. In general, men tend to have more muscle mass than women, and younger adults have more muscle mass than elderly adults.

The WHO classification was derived from studies of Europeans; thus, there has been subsequent discussion about creating further cutoff points for other ethnic populations. This push is mainly due to data that indicate that people with very low BMIs, particularly those of Asian descent, are at an increased risk for morbidity. A WHO expert consultation addressed this debate and considered whether population-specific cutoff points for BMI are necessary in this population. However, to date no conclusive data have suggested alternative cutoff points for people of Asian descent.[6]

Another consideration in the evaluation of overweight and obese individuals is weight distribution. Persons with central adiposity (also known as visceral, male pattern, android, or apple-shaped adiposity) may be at an increased risk for developing diseases, such as diabetes, even when these individuals fall within a normal BMI category. Males with a waist size greater than 40 inches and females with a waist size greater than 35 inches are at an increased risk for metabolic syndrome.[7]

Factors Contributing to Weight Gain and the Development of Diabetes: It is well recognized that as nations become more industrialized, the number of overweight and obese individuals increases. In addition to increases in body

Table **5.1**	Classifications for body mass index (BMI)
Classification	**BMI (kg/m^2)**
Underweight	<18.5
Normal weight	18.5–24.9
Overweight	25–29.9
Obesity class I	30–34.9
Obesity class II	35–39.9
Obesity class III (extreme)	≥40

From National Institutes of Health. The practical guide: identification, evaluation and treatment of overweight and obesity in adults. October, 2000. NIH Publication No 00-4084. http://www.nhlbi.nih.gov/guidelines/obesity/practgde.htm. Accessed September 9, 2007.

weight, other comorbid conditions increase as well, including hypertension, diabetes, and heart disease, and so do other noncardiovascular ailments, such as cancer and arthritis. Weight gain and obesity result from a complex interaction between genes and the environment characterized by a long-term positive energy balance due to a sedentary lifestyle, excessive caloric consumption, or a combination of the two.[8]

In a cross-sectional study using nationally representative data of U.S. adults 20 years of age or older from the 1999–2002 National Health and Nutrition Examination Survey, dietary energy density, or caloric intake, was independently and significantly associated with higher BMIs in women (β = 0.44, 95% confidence interval [CI], 0.14, 0.73) and trended toward a significant association in men (β = 0.37, 95% CI −0.007, 0.74, p = 0.054). Dietary energy density was associated with higher waist circumferences in both women (β = 1.11, 95% CI 0.42, 1.80) and men (β = 1.33, 95% CI 0.46, 2.19). Furthermore, dietary energy density was also independently associated with elevated fasting insulin levels (β = 0.65, 95% CI 0.18, 1.12) and metabolic syndrome (prevalence ratio = 1.10, 95% CI 1.03, 1.17).[9]

Metabolic Syndrome: Metabolic syndrome is a multifaceted syndrome characterized by the presence of three or more of the following: abdominal adiposity, hypertriglyceridemia, low high-density lipoprotein (HDL; the "good cholesterol"), hypertension, and an elevated fasting glucose. Metabolic syndrome is also known as syndrome X, dysmetabolic syndrome, insulin resistance syndrome, Reaven's syndrome, or **C**oronary Artery Disease, **H**ypertension, **A**dult Onset Diabetes (Typed), **O**besity and **S**troke (Australia).[10] Patients with metabolic syndrome are at a high risk for developing cardiovascular disease and diabetes. The primary causative factors are central adiposity or obesity and insulin resistance.

The constellation of factors contributing to this syndrome has been noted in the medical literature since the 1920s; however, with the advent of the second-generation atypical antipsychotics, this topic has been in the forefront of the medical literature once again.[11] Although the term was first coined in the 1970s by Haller, a German physician, the primary person associated with the theory of the metabolic syndrome is Gerald M. Reaven, an endocrinologist and professor emeritus at Stanford University in California.[12,13]

Table 5.2 depicts the criteria necessary to diagnose a patient with metabolic syndrome One should keep in mind that only three of the five "metabolic" criteria are necessary to meet the diagnosis of metabolic syndrome.

Partly due to the fact that individuals who suffer from schizophrenia have a higher risk of obesity and diabetes, and partly due to the fact that second-generation atypical antipsychotics increase the risk of obesity, hypertriglyceridemia, and diabetes, the incidence of metabolic syndrome is extremely high among patients with schizophrenia. According to the National Institutes of Mental Health–sponsored Clinical Antipsychotic Trials of Intervention Effectiveness (CATIE), the prevalence of metabolic syndrome among patients

Table **5.2**	Diagnostic criteria for the metabolic syndrome
Risk factor[a]	**Criteria**
Abdominal Obesity	Waist circumference[b]
Men	>102 cm (>40 in)
Women	>88 cm (>35 in)
Triglycerides	≥150 mg/dL, or
	On medication to treat elevated triglycerides
HDL cholesterol	
Men	<40 mg/dL
Women	<50 mg/dL, or
	On medication to treat low HDL
Blood pressure	Systolic ≥130 mm Hg, or
	Diastolic ≥85 mm Hg, or
	On medication to treat hypertension
Fasting glucose	≥100 mg/dl, or
	On medication to lower blood glucose

[a]Note: Patients must satisfy *three of the five* risk factors to meet the diagnosis for metabolic syndrome.
[b]Measured with a tape measure in a horizontal plane around the abdomen at level of iliac crest. Data from Grundy SM. Metabolic syndrome scientific statement by the American Heart Association and the National Heart, Lung, and Blood Institute. *Arterioscl Thromb Vasc Biol.* 2005;25:2243–2244.

with schizophrenia is 42.7%. Compared to individuals from the National Health and Nutrition Examination Survey III (NHANES), men and women with schizophrenia have two and three times the risk, respectively, of metabolic syndrome vs. those without schizophrenia.[14]

Challenges in Treating the Mentally Ill

Eating patterns of individuals are largely determined by the way in which they were raised, their family and others that surround them, social factors, and cultural influences. For most people, patterns that develop tend to remain constant throughout their lives. These enduring patterns are notoriously difficult to alter. Motivation has been found to be a key contributing factor necessary to successfully overcome these engrained patterns to achieve a health goal through proper nutrition.[15]

Symptomatology: In addition to the direct negative metabolic impact that many psychotropic drugs possess, one must also consider other added challenges present in mentally ill people, including symptomatology (e.g., anhedonia, hopelessness, thought disorganization, decreased energy, difficulty with concentration, decreased social interaction, depression, paranoia, negative symptoms) that make it difficult to focus, learn, and retain information. In addition, the side effects of medications (e.g., sedation, confusion, drowsiness) may also negatively affect outcomes and motivation. These may provide further challenges when trying to educate patients.

Patients with schizophrenia prove to be especially challenging, because profound negative symptoms affect interest and motivation with regard to health and well-being.[16] Compounding this with the presence of delusions and hallucinations in patients with poorly controlled illness and thought disorganization further complicates this problem. All of these factors make it challenging to implement strict dietary program in this population.

Patients with depression or bipolar depression may lack interest in their well-being and suffer from difficulty maintaining focus. Furthermore, many depressed patients suffer from decreased energy, psychomotor retardation, and changes in appetite, which may further promote weight gain. All of these make it very challenging to successfully implement a weight loss program in depressed patients.

Patients with bipolar disorder who are manic suffer from racing thoughts, distractibility, and agitation, making it very challenging for these patients to focus and learn. One can clearly see the many challenges this would present in educating patients with poorly controlled mania.

In addition, many patients with mental illnesses such as depression, bipolar depression, or schizophrenia with strong negative symptoms, often state that eating is one of the few highlights of their day. Dieticians must work hard to teach patients that proper eating can be rewarding, and that they can still eat many of the foods they associate with pleasure—just in limited amounts.

Ultimately, the cognitive functioning level of people with mental illness may determine the appropriate level of intensity of education about diabetes nutrition. Although a particular patient may not be suitable for education, a family member, friend, or a caregiver who is interested in playing an active role in the patient's care may be encouraged to participate in educational instruction by the dietician.

Social Factors: Other factors that come into play when treating the mentally ill are social factors. Often, people afflicted with mental illness have limited financial resources that may affect their ability to select healthy, less calorie-dense foods. Many eat at fast food restaurants or pick up calorie-dense foods from convenience stores. Furthermore, financial resources are necessary to access exercise equipment or a gymnasium, as well as to pay for dietary counseling and education.

Many mentally ill patients often reside in board-and-care facilities. This may present challenges with regards to a patient's diet as well. To make a profit and stay in business, operators of board-and-care homes face strong economic pressures to reduce operating expenses. Among these costs is the cost of food. Many times snacks are donated from nearby restaurants, and high-calorie baked goods are far too abundant, because they require no preparation, have a long shelf life, and are extremely filling. Patients living in board-and-care facilities have few meal choices, making it difficult for patients to change what they eat. Often there are limited amounts fruits and vegetables available, because they spoil rapidly and can be expensive. Board-and-care facilities often provide many calorie-dense meals and snacks with little nutritional value. The meals are often filled with an abundance of saturated fat. It is common for board-and-care operators to provide large portions of starchy foods with all daily meals, such as potatoes and breads, because these are both filling and easy to prepare for the masses. Unfortunately, these provide little nutritional value and are far too calorie dense. Despite the restrictions of food choices, dieticians can still assist patients by teaching proper food selection from what is available and enforcing portion control.

Interventions

With appropriate assistance, it is possible to help patients prevent or manage their weight through proper diet and exercise, as well as appropriate pharmacologic management. There are many means available to assist patients in managing their weight, glucose, lipids, and blood pressure. Health care providers are encouraged to work together as a team to develop the best treatment plan for an individual patient, one which is aggressive enough to reduce cardiovascular risk factors, but also acceptable for the patient to adhere to. Psychiatrists must work closely with endocrinologists, internists, dieticians, and pharmacists, as well as patients and their caregivers, to develop an optimal, patient-specific care plan.

Nonpharmacologic Treatment: Contrary to the challenges faced, many studies have successfully demonstrated weight loss in the mentally ill. Most successful programs consist of three key components: 1) implementation of a low-fat, low-calorie diet, 2) increased physical activity, and 3) behavioral therapy. Taken together, these factors have been shown to be successful in promoting weight loss among patients treated with typical antipsychotics[17–21] or atypical antipsychotics.[5,15,22–28]

In one such study. Centorrino et al. illustrated that weight loss obtained during the initial months of the intervention was largely sustained up to 48 weeks later, even during less intensive follow-up.[5] A study by O'Keefe demonstrated that patients with antipsychotic-associated weight gain are able to lose approximately half of their initial weight gain through dietary and behavioral interventions.[28] Even in patients taking psychotropic agents most notorious for weight gain, such as olanzapine, behavioral and dietary interventions have still been proven to result in successful weight loss.[23,24,27]

Diet and exercise not only help to maintain proper weight, but they also help manage glucose control, improve lipid profiles, and maintain blood pressure. Recognizing the potential for development of weight gain and obesity is key to preventing the problem before it happens. It has been noted that weight gain usually occurs within the first few months of antipsychotic treatment.[29] Fortunately, early behavioral interventions have been shown to help attenuate antipsychotic-induced weight gain in the drug-naïve new-onset population.[26] Thus, one should not wait to implement interventions early on in treatment. Early referral to a qualified nutrition professional on starting a patient on medication with weight gain potential is optimal.

Although many of the patients in published studies accomplished only small weight losses, it is necessary to keep in mind that even minimal changes in body weight, as low as 5%, have been shown to result in clinically meaningful reductions in morbidity and mortality, including significantly lowering the risk of diabetes mellitus, hypertension, and hyperlipidemia.[30,31]

Diet There have been many successful weight management programs applied to both patients with schizophrenia and bipolar disorder.[5,15,17,18,20,22–27,28,32–40] All of the studies showed either more weight loss in the intervention group or less weight gain than in nonintervention group. Later studies also showed improvement in outcomes relating to metabolic syndrome.[5,15,25,27]

The earliest inpatient studies focused primarily on caloric restriction.[17,18,20,32–34] Significant amounts of weight loss were achieved, although there were noteworthy limitations to the applicability of these interventions. The participants were studied in a controlled environment (they were inpatients); thus, the element of choice of foods was essentially removed. One must also keep in mind that these studies took place prior to the availability of the second-generation antipsychotics.

In the past 20 years, the focus has shifted to outpatient management and interventions. Many strategies have been used in these studies to help patients achieve caloric restriction. Most involved sessions with a dietician to assist the patient in making better food choices and encouraging increased caloric expenditure through regular exercise. A few of the studies encouraged patients to use a diary to monitor daily food intake and/or exercise.[15,27] The process of documenting food intake can serve two means. It is educational with regard to proper food choices, and it serves as a deterrent to prevent overeating.

One of the recent prospective randomized controlled trials based on a simple eating plan, the "Stoplight Diet," was very effective.[26] This diet was originally developed for children by Leonard H. Epstein in the 1970s.[40] The diet teaches proper nutrition by linking foods to the three signals on a traffic light: high-calorie foods are depicted as "red" and should be eaten rarely (e.g., desserts, pastries, fast foods, fried and cream-based foods); moderate-calorie foods are "yellow" and can be eaten in moderation (e.g., eggs, low-fat dairy products, breads and other grain products, meats, poultry and fish); and low-calorie foods are "green" and can be eaten freely (e.g., plain vegetables, fresh fruit, and low- or no-calorie beverages).

Regardless of the technique used in the later studies, common principles applied helped patients to choose healthier, lower calorie foods. Weight gain is caused by a positive energy balance or, when energy in (i.e., ingested) is greater than energy out (i.e., expended). Thus, the goal is to teach patients to control their caloric intake by decreasing calorie-dense foods and moderating portion sizes. In this way, patients can reverse the positive energy balance. When implementing a dietary plan, a good rule of thumb is that a calorie deficit of 500 to 1000 kcal/day less than the patient's baseline intake should be implemented.[4] This roughly equates to a total daily intake of 1000 to 1200 kcal/day for women and 1200 to 1500 kcal/day for men. This reduced calorie intake alone can be expected to produce a 1- to 2-pound weight loss per week. In addition, one should strive to keep total daily fat intake to less than 30%.

The first step in dietary counseling is to discern what a person consumes regularly with regard to meals and fluids. Often, patients taking antipsychotics or antidepressants describe regular consumption of sodas and juices to self-treat the anticholinergic-associated dry mouth caused by their medication. Excessive caffeinated soda intake is also common, in an effort to combat drowsiness associated with their medication. If a patient drinks soda or juice regularly, the first step is to encourage drinking water instead. The simplicity of the first approach gradually moves toward more complicated alterations in other aspects of the diet, as the patient illustrates gradual adherence toward each goal. Meeting goals helps instill a feeling of success in the patient, which helps encourage the patient to meet more goals in the future.

The second major technique used to promote the experience of success is to provide patients with a means to analyze their own eating patterns and progress. This can be accomplished by keeping daily food and exercise diaries. Over time, patients begin to express their realization of problem habits during their appointments with the dietician. The dietician addresses these acknowledgments and gives positive feedback along with an explanation of how to take precautions not to gain the weight back. Patients feel rewarded in knowing that they are playing a part in their treatment program.

As with any population, it is crucial to educate patients about making healthier choices. Often, patients have limited selections for foods; thus dieticians must educate patients with regard to proper food selection at fast food restaurants and convenience stores. Patients can be advised to place a slightly smaller portion of food on their plate, eat only what is there, and then wait 20 minutes to assess fullness. This is done to avoid extra caloric intake via grazing.

In addition to portion control, small changes such as proper food selections can add up to substantial differences. For example, patients can help by using mustard instead of mayonnaise; eating whole wheat bread instead of white bread; consuming oatmeal and whole grain cereals instead of sugary cereals; refraining from salad dressings (choose 1 tablespoon olive oil and vinegar instead); taking the skin off chicken; and choosing more foods that are baked, grilled, or roasted, instead of fried. Dieticians can also review with patients healthier alternatives at fast food restaurants, such as salads with low-calorie dressing or baked chicken.

To facilitate adherence, cultural, ethnic, and financial considerations must all be taken into consideration. One must be creative in developing teaching tools that match the level of the patient's understanding and his or her educational background.[41,42] For example, if a patient cannot read, a more visual basic such as food models may need to be used. In addition, an "American" diet of white rice, vegetables, and chicken (breast) may be very unfamiliar to a Hispanic person who is used to eating rice, beans, and tortillas.

There are many different types of dietary interventions currently being used by dieticians. The important thing to keep in mind is that every patient's health status is constantly changing. Reevaluations and adjustments in the treatment plan should occur regularly throughout a patient's lifetime. Patients must be given the tools necessary to achieve positive outcomes and they must be provided constant support and encouragement. Necessary learning tools include information on diet and nutrition, physical activity, and behavioral techniques.

Dietary Goals in Patients With Diabetes
Diabetes is a chronic and progressive disease. The goal of nutrition in the diabetic patient is to assist the patient in achieving superior glycemic control to prevent or delay micro- and macrovascular complications while minimizing hyperglycemia and controlling weight.[43] The results of the United Kingdom Prospective Diabetes Studies (UKPDS) and Diabetes Control and Complications Trial (DCCT) indicate that tight control of blood glucose (and blood pressure in type 2 diabetes) can prevent or delay the long-term complications of diabetes.[43,44] Food choices, particularly carbohydrate intake, are directly related to blood glucose. Thus, management of carbohydrate intake is of utmost importance and should be strongly emphasized along with blood glucose monitoring, appropriate pharmacotherapy, and physical activity for optimal outcomes.

Many people with diabetes have both high blood glucose and blood pressure levels, and these patients are particularly at risk for diabetic complications. The UKPDS support previous guidelines and suggest one should aim for near-normal glucose levels, a glycosylated hemoglobin A_{1c} value less than 7%, and tight blood pressure control.[44] This glycemic target can be reached by a combination of oral agents and/or insulin therapy along with diet. The UKPDS also emphasizes the importance of controlling other cardiovascular risk factors, such as cholesterol and smoking.[44] The study attempts to emphasize the fact that overall cardiovascular risk needs to be reduced. In other words, the goal in managing diabetes no longer just involves blood glucose control, but rather centers on the reduction of all of the cardiovascular risk factors.

The first step in developing a nutritional plan is a thorough assessment of the individual's nutritional status, their usual and customary food intake, as well as expenditures. Baseline measurements include height, weight, calculation of BMI, a measurement of body fat distribution (waist measurement), assessment of physical activity, medical history, review of current laboratory data, an assessment of psychosocial and economic issues, and the patient's educational level and their ability to learn. Monitoring and assessments should be ongoing throughout the patient's lifespan and should be outcome driven. Outcome markers, such as blood glucose levels, A_{1c}, blood lipids, blood pressure, renal status, and weight and waist size, are important assessment parameters that influence the management plan.[45]

There is no such thing as a "diabetic" diet. Meals need to be well-balanced, offer plenty of color (i.e., fruits and vegetables), and be fiber-rich. Presently, priority is given to the total amount of carbohydrates consumed at each meal or snack, rather than the source of the carbohydrate. Most patients with diabetes can tolerate at least 30 grams of carbohydrates per meal (or at least two exchanges); less than 30 grams per meal is not recommended and can be harmful, especially for patients who are taking sulfonylureas or insulin and who are susceptible to hypoglycemia.[41]

The goal of diet is not only to maintain normal glucose levels, but also to help to improve cholesterol and blood pressure, as well as to maintain normal body weight. All of these together will aid to prevent long term complications. In addition, even a modest weight loss can make a significant difference in blood glucose and lipids, thus weight loss should be encouraged in those who are overweight.

Recommended Caloric Distribution for Patients With Diabetes Protein intake should comprise approximately 10% to 20% of the daily caloric intake. There is no solid evidence that a higher protein intake (>20% of calories) contributes to the development of nephropathy; however, with signs of microalbuminuria (indicative of glomerular injury), a protein intake of less than 0.8 g/kg/day or approximately 10% of the daily calorie requirements may delay the progression of renal failure.[46] Any further restriction in protein may result in malnutrition and muscle weakness. One should keep in mind that protein requirements are increased during illness, infection, or surgery.[47]

If dietary protein contributes 10% to 20% of the total daily calories, the remaining 80% to 90% of calories should be distributed between fat and carbohydrate. Blood glucose and insulin response are influenced by both the source, simple or complex, and amount of carbohydrate consumed. Therefore, daily carbohydrate intake should range from 45% to 60% of total calories, with total fat calories kept under 30%, and specifically, less than 7% of calories should come from saturated fats.[48]

The distribution of monounsaturated fats and carbohydrates should be individualized based on a nutrition assessment and realistic goals. The levels estimated for these nutrients should reflect desired blood glucose levels, lipids, and weight. If weight loss is a primary concern, adjusting total energy to facilitate weight loss combined with decreasing dietary fat to 25% to 30% of total energy can be an effective approach. Fiber intake also comes into play,

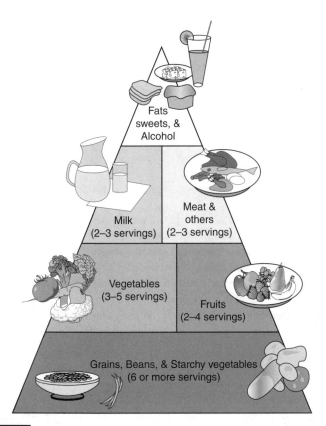

Figure **5.1**   Diabetes food pyramid. From http://ndep.nih.gov/diabetes/
MealPlanner/pyramid.htm.

in that soluble fiber has a minor effect on inhibiting blood glucose absorption
from the small intestine.[49]

Diabetes Food Pyramid   The Diabetes Food Guide Pyramid can be a practical
teaching tool for people with diabetes (Figure 5.1). The pyramid can be
described as a "starting point" for nutrition management of diabetes by indicating the number of servings per day and appropriate serving size for food
groups. These tools can also provide the basis for introducing the concept of
carbohydrate counting by helping patients begin to recognize which groups
certain foods fall under and by giving patients an idea about the recommended
proportion for intake (related to the size of the piece in the pyramid).

Plate Method for Patients With Diabetes   One of the easiest ways to teach
individuals with diabetes about diet is to utilize the "plate method," a visual

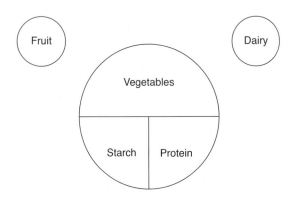

Figure **5.2**   **The Plate Method (based on a 9-inch pie plate). One-half plate = nonstarchy vegetables (e.g., salad, broccoli, spinach, bell peppers); one-fourth plate = carbohydrates (e.g., bread, noodles, rice, corn, potatoes, or fruit); one-fourth plate = protein (e.g., poultry, fish, seafood, or red meat). One should also include a small side dish of fruit and dairy product like a glass of low or non-fat milk or some low fat cheese. Data from American Diabetes Association Diabetes Learning Center, http://www.diabetes.org/all-about-diabetes/chan_eng/i3/i3p4.htm.**

learning aid developed by the American Diabetes Association (ADA). This visual learning aid uses the image of a round plate divided into three sections One quarter of the plate should be filled with protein, the second quarter with carbohydrates, and the other half with nonstarchy vegetables (Figure 5.2).[50] Therefore, without delving into the complexities of calorie or carbohydrate counting, a person is able to create a balanced meal that is less calorie-dense. This allows patients to eat what they like and helps maintain proper portion levels.

Exchange Lists for Patients With Diabetes   Exchange lists for meal planning offer an organized approach to meal planning for people with diabetes (Table 5.3).[50] When using the exchange/choice lists, the dietician should ensure that the person has a full understanding of how to read the exchange chart. Exchange lists are foods grouped together by caloric similarity. Each serving of a food has about the same amount of carbohydrate, protein, and fat, as well as calories, as other foods on the list. Thus, any food on the list can be "exchanged" or traded for any other food on the same list. Foods are listed with their serving sizes, which are typically measured after cooking. For example, a slice of bread can be traded or "exchanged" for one-half cup of cooked cereal. Each of these foods equals one starch choice.

Table 5.3	Exchange groups			
Group/lists	Carbohydrate (g)	Protein (g)	Fat (g)	Calories
Carbohydrate groups				
Starch	15	3	0–1	80
Fruit	15			60
Milk[a]				
Fat free/low fat	12	8	0–3	90
Reduced	12	8	5	120
Whole	12	7	8	150
Other carbohydrates	15	Varies	Varies	Varies
Nonstarchy vegetable	5	2	—	25
Meat and meat substitute group				
Very lean	—	3	0–1	35
Lean	—	7	3	55
Medium-fat	—	7	5	75
High-fat	—	7	8	45
Fat Group	—	—	—	45

[a]Fat free milk is recommended.
Directions: Patients are given exchange lists of foods from their dietician. Patients then have the freedom to select from various food options in the exchange lists. For example, one piece of bread falls under the "starch" category and has 15 g of carbohydrates, 3 g of protein, and 0 to 1 g of fat. If the patient does not favor bread, he or she may select another starch, for example, 1/3 cup of cooked rice, which contains the same amount of carbohydrates, protein, and fat, and thus the same calories.
Exchange lists may be ordered from the American Diabetes Association (ADA) by calling (800)-DIABETES, or (800) 342-2383.
Data from American Diabetes Association Diabetes Learning Center. http://www.diabetes.org/all-about-diabetes/chan_eng/i3/i3p4.htm. Accessed May 6, 2007.

In the beginning, patients need to measure the size of each serving until they can successfully "eyeball" the correct serving size. Most patients with diabetes benefit from having 30 to 45 grams of carbohydrate (or two to four exchanges) per meal. The most accurate way to determine whether they are receiving too much or too little carbohydrate is by monitoring the patient's blood sugar trends.

Carbohydrate Counting in Diabetes The rationale for carbohydrate counting is that carbohydrates are the main factor affecting postprandial blood glucose levels. Although this technique emphasizes the importance of the total amount of carbohydrates rather than the source, the protein and fat contribution to total energy intake cannot be disregarded. The advantage of this technique includes flexible food choices and a single nutrient focus, which helps simplify matters. People using this technique should be motivated and knowledgeable regarding the basic concepts of meal planning, the carbohydrate content of foods, and blood glucose monitoring.

At the basic level of carbohydrate counting (level 1), the patient and dietician determine the total amount of carbohydrates that will be consumed per meal or snack. This is based on the person's usual carbohydrate intake of foods. Once the goal for the carbohydrate intake is established, the person learns to determine the amount of carbohydrates in different portion sizes of carbohydrate-containing foods in an effort to count his or her carbohydrate intake. As the person becomes more skilled in carbohydrate counting, he or she may be ready to take on the challenges of advanced forms of carbohydrate counting: pattern management and carbohydrate-to-insulin ratio. Advanced carbohydrate counting requires special skills and considerations. Pattern management involves working with the healthcare team to find patterns in blood sugar levels that relate to diet, diabetes medications, and physical activity. If the person is taking multiple daily injections of insulin or using an insulin pump, learning about carbohydrate-to-insulin ratios allows the patient to make adjustments in insulin dose based upon the amount of carbohydrate that is eaten.[50]

Blood Sugar Monitoring   In order for health care providers to best assist their patients, it is imperative that patients check and record their blood sugars routinely so that adjustments can be made. As patients keep track of these numbers, they can begin to discover trends in their glucose levels and discover how various foods and the presence or lack of physical activity can affect fasting plasma glucose levels. It is essential that patients are able to recognize signs and symptoms of hypoglycemia and how to correct them with the proper amount of carbohydrate, particularly when changes are being made to a patient's diet.

Patients typically begin to experience signs and symptoms of low blood sugar when blood glucose levels fall below 70 mg/dL. Symptoms of hypoglycemia can include hunger, nervousness, weakness, shakiness, chest palpitations, sweating, and dizziness. However, some patients oftentimes do not perceive the symptoms of hypoglycemia, particularly those with a long history of diabetes or those taking beta blockers. The ability to sense low blood glucose can be affected by the duration of diabetes and the rate at which the blood glucose falls. Severe hypoglycemia can lead to loss of consciousness or coma.

In general, when a patient's blood sugar falls below 70 mg/dL, he or she can enact the "rule of 15/15" by taking 15 grams of glucose (e.g., one-half cup of orange juice, one-half cup regular soda, three to four candies such as Life Savers, or three to four glucose tablets) and wait 15 minutes before retesting the blood sugar. If the blood sugar is still less than 70 mg/dL, patients should intake another 15 grams of glucose. Once the blood sugar is more than 70 mg/dL, patients should complete the treatment by eating a snack that contains carbohydrate, fat and protein, such as one-half of a peanut butter sandwich or a few crackers and a glass of low-fat or nonfat milk.

Exercise Regular exercise is beneficial for the majority of people with diabetes; it promotes the expenditure of calories, cardiovascular fitness, muscle building (which burns fat), weight loss, and a healthy lipoprotein profile.[51,52] The last is particularly important for persons with diabetes, because they are at an increased risk for cardiovascular disease. Regular exercise is beneficial in the prevention or correction of atherosclerotic cardiovascular disease by improving the HDL/LDL ratio. Regular exercise can improve body composition by decreasing body fat and increasing muscle mass, which further enhances insulin sensitivity and glucose metabolism. Routine exercise can assist in weight reduction efforts by helping reverse the positive energy balance.[51]

Increasing physical activity can be accomplished in several ways: simply increasing normal daily physical activity by participating in household chores or choosing walking as an alternative to driving or taking the elevator, as well as implementing a routine exercise program. An exercise program should start gradually, for example, walking 10 minutes a day for three days a week. However, ultimately the goal is to increase the duration of exercise up to 30 to 45 minutes per day for most days of the week. Exercise programs should incorporate activities that are appealing to the patient, such as bowling, swimming, or bicycling.

Behavioral Interventions The third component in a weight loss plan is behavioral therapy. Behavior therapy provides patients with a set of principles and techniques with which to modify eating and activity habits. It typically consists of self-monitoring, goal setting, and stimulus control. Cognitive therapy focuses more on problem solving and cognitive restructuring to achieve changes.[52] Dieticians often use behavioral interventions when developing dietary programs for patients. It is clear that the most successful outpatient programs, defined by successful weight loss and a reduction of markers of the metabolic syndrome, are multimodal in nature, incorporating behavioral interventions, nutritional counseling, and a structured exercise program.

One of the common elements in most of the successful weight loss studies throughout the years is the use of behavioral therapy or cognitive-behavioral therapy. Studies have shown that behavioral interventions, when used in conjunction with diet and exercise interventions, promote larger weight losses than diet and exercise alone.[53] Behavioral strategies include self-monitoring (e.g., food diaries), cognitive restructuring (identifying any false perceptions the patient may have that could undermine weight loss efforts), stimulus control (identifying "cues" that trigger overeating and developing techniques to prevent this from happening), social support (involving family members or caregivers in the weight loss program, or participating in group programs), stress management (relaxation techniques and coping strategies), and a reward system (providing a small reward for each goal achieved).[4]

Patients' motivation is stimulated when they experience immediate and continued success. Such success can be measured in numbers, such as pounds of weight loss or total daily calories. Small, nonoverwhelming goals should be set together by the patient and the dietician and measured frequently. New goals should be added slowly and only when the patient has successfully met their initial goals first. In this manner, patients are more inclined to continue the newly learned behavior, and as a result, they continue to lose more weight over time.

Food diaries are a tool that can be used to provide the patient with a means to analyze and assess their own eating habits and progress over time. Tracking dietary choices and linking these to positive outcomes can assist the patient in understanding what works best for them. In addition, it can assist dieticians in assessing why things are or are not working. Frequent visits and reinforcement help patients to stay within their prescribed nutrition guidelines and continue on a positive path toward progressive weight loss.

Stages of Change Model   It is important to assist patients in understanding their health to help them make changes. When counseled by a dietician, patients seem to understand lifestyle alterations, but consistent lifelong behavior changes pose a challenge to most. Behavior change has come to become understood as a process of identifiable stages through which patient passes. Understanding the process provides health care professionals with the additional tools to assist patients, who are often discouraged and not motivated.[54] The stages of change model shows that, for most individuals, a change in behavior occurs gradually, with the patient moving from being uninterested, unaware, or unwilling to make a change (precontemplation), to considering a change (contemplation), to deciding and preparing to make a change.[54] Genuine, determined action is then undertaken by the patient and over time, attempts are made to maintain the new behavior. Relapses are inevitable and become part of the process of working toward a life-long change.[54]

It is imperative for the dietician to assess patients correctly and place them into the appropriate stage according to this model, and to facilitate the patient along the stages of change.[54] Once this stage has been determined, the health care professional can proceed with a plan that is appropriate for the individual. If the patient starts to resist, this is evidence that the health care professional has moved too far ahead of the patient in the process, and that a shift back to empathy and thought-provoking questions is required.[54] Some patients may be quite ambitious and some may be at risk for feeling stressed or overwhelmed. It is the health care professional's job to make sure that any risk of anxiety be avoided due to the risk of creating an aversion to any possible changes.

Surgical Intervention At this time weight loss surgery, either vertical banded gastroplasty or Roux-en-Y gastric bypass, is the most effective weight loss alternative for patients with obesity and morbid obesity in the general population in whom traditional methods of diet, exercise, and behavioral interventions fail. Unfortunately, the presence of psychiatric illness may serve as a barrier to selection for these surgeries. The International Federation for the Surgery of Obesity states that one of the widely accepted criteria for selection of a candidate is that the patient has "no psychiatric illness or drug dependency."[55] Nonetheless, there are currently no set guidelines on what specific disorders should be eliminated from consideration, and practices vary widely.[56] In a recent study of the prevalence of psychiatric disorders in bariatric surgery candidates, over half had a lifetime history of an Axis I disorder, and approximately one third met diagnostic criteria for Axis I and II disorders.[57]

There is very limited data available with regards to outcomes from weight loss surgery in patients with mental illness. A small study was conducted looking at five patients with well-controlled schizophrenia and morbid obesity versus individuals with morbid obesity without mental illness. Six months after bariatric surgery, both groups had comparable weight loss.[58] To date there are no longer term studies to evaluate weight loss in the mentally ill following bariatric surgery. Clearly further studies are warranted before any definitive recommendations can be made with regard to surgically managing patients with obesity and concurrent schizophrenia or other mental illnesses.

Pharmacological Interventions

Proper Psychotropic Selection Before starting a patient on a psychotropic medication, it is always necessary to take into account the patient's metabolic risk factors at baseline, along with his or her family history of metabolic disorders. The clinician should always carefully weigh the pros and cons of each individual psychotropic medication, and should consider choosing a medication that minimally affects weight gain, glucose, and lipids. If a patient develops metabolic complications secondary to treatment with a specific psychotropic, one option is to attempt to change to another medication. However, this is not always feasible. More often than not, attempts must be made to manage the metabolic complications through nonpharmacologic interventions (diet, exercise, and behavioral interventions) and by using additional medications such as oral hypoglycemics and/or insulin, lipid lowering agents, antihypertensives, and weight loss agents.

Pharmacological Agents For those patients without mental illness who have a BMI $\geq$30 kg/m^2, or for those with a BMI $\geq$27 kg/m^2 with additional cardiovascular comorbidities who fail to lose 8% to 10% of their baseline body weight after 6 months of interventions, the clinician would typically consider the addition of a weight loss agent.[4] Choices would include agents that help suppress appetite by increasing serotonin, norepinephrine, and/or dopamine (e.g., mazindol, phentermine, chlorphentermine, diethylpropion, sibutramine), agents that increase metabolic rate (e.g., stimulants such as caffeine and ephedrine), or those which inhibit the absorption of dietary fat (e.g., orlistat).[4] Average weight loss in the short term (less than 6 months) with any of these agents has been reported to range from 4 to 20 pounds.[4] One should note that these agents are recommended to be used only in the short term. There have been no long-term studies with these agents.

Unfortunately, there have been very few studies of weight loss agents in patients with mental illness. Furthermore, none of the available anorexiant agents currently on the market has been specifically approved for use in the mentally ill. Furthermore, many of the available agents that work by increasing norepinephrine and serotonin may potentially interact with antidepressants and antipsychotics. In addition, there is concern that centrally acting anorexiants could potentially exacerbate psychosis in patients with schizophrenia. For these reasons, the clinician should always focus on the standard triad for weight loss (diet, exercise, and behavioral interventions) before resorting to pharmacological interventions in the mentally ill.

The literature on nonanorexiant agents to promote weight loss in the psychiatric population is relatively scarce. Medications such as amantadine, reboxetine, nizatidine, famotidine, fluoxetine, and topiramate have been studied with mostly disappointing results.[59–68] Perhaps the most promising study thus far has been with metformin. Results from an open-label study of pediatric patients who experienced more than a 10% weight gain on an atypical antipsychotic or valproic acid showed statistically significant decreases in both weight and BMI with metformin 500 mg three times daily, without concurrent dietary or exercise interventions.[69] However, when one takes into consideration the fact that larger prospective trials have shown that dietary and lifestyle interventions resulted in statistically significantly more weight loss compared with metformin-treated patients, these results seem far less significant.[70]

The data on anorexiant agents in the mentally ill is even more scarce. Phenylpropanolamine failed to promote weight loss in one study of patients on clozapine, as did chlorphentermine and phenmetrazine.[21,71] Sibutramine has been the most studied of the anorexiant agents with efficacy reported in olanzapine-treated patients but not clozapine-treated patients.[72,73] However, one must consider the fact that this is a centrally acting agent that affects serotonin and can potentially result in changes in mood and it may interact with other psychotropic medications.

Perhaps the safest weight loss agent in the psychiatric population is orlistat, because it works peripherally, not centrally. However, to date, orlistat has rarely been studied in the mentally ill, and currently only case reports support use of this agent.[74,75] Orlistat may inhibit the absorption of fat-soluble vitamins, and side effects include fecal urgency, flatulence, and oily spotting, particularly if the patient fails to maintain a fat-restricted diet. Thus, dietary counseling is a necessary component that must be used in conjunction with this agent.

Resources

Because referral to a dietician is not always feasible, there are steps that a primary health care provider can take to assist their patients with weight management. *The Practical Guide: Identification, Evaluation, and Treatment of Overweight and Obesity in Adults*, developed jointly by the National Heart, Lung, and Blood Institute (NHLBI) and the North American Association for the Study of Obesity (NAASO), is one such guide. This guide is available for download for free online at http://www.nhlbi.nih.gov/guidelines/obesity/practgde.htm.[76] It contains useful information for health care providers and patients with regard to weight loss, diet, and exercise. The publication presents sample low-calorie menus; healthy alternatives to high-fat or sugary foods; exchange lists; typical calorie content breakdowns of common foods from a number of different cultural backgrounds; sample exercise programs; as well as diaries to chart weight, physical activity, and daily food intake.

The *2005 Dietary Guidelines for Americans* [www.health.gov/dietaryguidelines/] is a valuable resource on basic nutrition guidelines to improve health. Here, one can find many free downloadable brochures available for professionals and patients. In addition to the general guidelines about eating habits and exercise, www.mypyramid.gov includes an interactive section which allows one to customize a nutrition regimen according to age, gender, height, weight, and physical activity. The pyramid concept is based on the Food Guide Pyramid from 1992 which groups foods into categories such as grains, beans, vegetables, fruits, milk, and meats. Each portion of the pyramid is sized according to the amount the individual person should consume.

Helpful Online Sources:
American Diabetes Association Diabetes Learning Center—www.diabetes.org/all-about-diabetes/chan_eng/i3/i3p4.htm
American Association of Diabetes Educators—www.aadenet.org
American Diabetes Association—www.ada.org
American Dietetic Association—www.eatright.org
Dietary Guidelines for Americans—www.health.gov/dietaryguidelines
Idaho's Plate Method—www.platemethod.com
My Food Pyramid—www.mypyramid.gov
Voice of the Diabetic—www.nfb.org/diabetes.htm

Basic Nutrition Concepts:
Often, psychiatrists end up managing many of the ailments of the psychiatrically ill, not only the psychiatric disorder, but all of the associated comorbid illnesses—diabetes, hyperlipidemia, hypertension, and obesity. As a result, it is becoming necessary for psychiatrists to maintain a solid knowledge base of nutrition and diet.

In general, there are three sources of calories from food: fats, proteins, and carbohydrates. It is recommended that the average person maintain a diet that consists of less than 30% from fats, 10% to 15% from protein, and 40% to

60% from carbohydrates. In addition to these caloric requirements, fiber is required to maintain gastrointestinal regulation. Other requirements include various vitamins and minerals. The following terms and definitions are useful in assisting with reviewing basic nutrition concepts.

Calorie–Technically the kilocalorie, but referred to as a "calorie," this is a unit of measurement of energy derived from food. The biochemical calorie is a unit of energy that raises 1 kg of water by 1 degree Celsius. Other countries use the joule or kilojoule.

Carbohydrate–Carbohydrates contribute four calories per gram of weight. Carbohydrates are usually classified as simple carbohydrates, such as table sugar, or complex carbohydrates, such as fruits, vegetables, and grains (e.g., rice). Carbohydrates come primarily from plant sources, with the exception of lactose, which comes from dairy products. The main function of carbohydrates is to provide energy for the body to use.

Cholesterol–Cholesterol is a fat-like substance that is made by the body and is also found naturally in foods from animal sources such as meat, fish, poultry, eggs, and dairy products. Foods high in cholesterol include liver and organ meats, egg yolks, and dairy fats. Cholesterol is carried in the bloodstream, and when levels are too high, it deposits onto the walls of the blood vessels. Over time, these deposits can build up, causing the blood vessels to narrow and blood flow to decrease, which increases the risk of heart disease.[77] It is recommended that the average person maintain an intake of less than less than 300 mg/day of cholesterol, or less for those individuals who suffer from hyperlipidemia.

Fat–Fat is the most calorie-dense of all of the macronutrients, contributing nine calories per gram of weight. It is recommended that less than 30% of people's diet comes from fat.[78] The types of fat are broken down as follows:

Saturated Fats–These fats are solid or nearly solid at room temperature. All animal fats (meat, poultry, and dairy) contain saturated fats. These fats can raise blood cholesterol levels, increasing the risk of heart disease. Current guidelines recommend that saturated fats be kept below 7% of total calories in the diet.[48]

Trans fats–Most trans fats are created through a manufacturing process that turns liquid oils into a solid fat, although small amounts are also naturally present in meat and dairy products. Trans fats behave like saturated fats, remaining solid at room temperature. Trans fats may raise LDL cholesterol levels while decreasing HDL cholesterol, which can increase the risk of heart disease. Recommendations are to keep total daily intake of trans fat to less than 2 grams/day.[78]

Polyunsaturated and monounsaturated fats–These fats are found in vegetable oils such as olive, canola, and soybean oils, as well as nuts. Omega-3 polyunsaturated fats are also found in seafood such as fish and shellfish. Replacing saturated fats with polyunsaturated fats helps maintain cardiovascular health.[78]

Fiber–Fiber is usually classified on food labels as a subset of carbohydrates. Fiber is a diverse group of compounds, including lignin and complex carbohydrates that cannot be digested by human enzymes in the small intestine.[79] Fiber is only found in plant sources such as whole grains, fruits, and vegetables. Some specialized fibers are used in food processing to thicken foods, such as guar gum and pectins. These contribute a small amount of fiber to non-plant foods. A fiber intake of at least 20 to 35 grams/day from a variety of food sources is recommended. Fiber helps maintain proper gastrointestinal regulation and decrease cholesterol reabsorption. Fiber also adds satiety by decreasing gastric emptying time.

Protein–Proteins contribute four calories per gram of weight. Protein rich foods include meats, chicken, fish, eggs, dairy products, and beans. Protein helps add a sense of satiety to a meal. The main function of protein is to help maintain support of our cells, organs and muscle.

Conclusion

When attempting to manage the multifaceted disorder known as metabolic syndrome, one must always take into account the challenges present in those who suffer from mental illness. Furthermore, it is important to emphasize that no single treatment plan should be expected to be the solution to a patient's well-being. It is essential to realize that the best results can be obtained only when one uses an integrative, collaborative, team approach to treatment by taking into consideration recommendations from the psychiatrist, internist, endocrinologist, pharmacist, dietician, caregiver, and most importantly, the patient.

References

1. National Center for Health Statistics Centers for Disease Control and Prevention. U.S. Department of Health and Human Services. Prevalence of obesity and overweight among adults: *Health* United States, 2003–2004. *E-Stats.* Cited March 31, 2007. http://www.cdc.gov/nchs/products/pubs/pubd/hestats/overweight/overwght_adult_03.htm.
2. Dickerson FB, Brown CH, Kreyenbuhl JA, et al. Obesity among individuals with serious mental illness. *Acta Psychiatr Scand.* 2006;113(4):306–313.
3. Weiden PJ, Mackell JA, McDonnell DD. Obesity as a risk factor for antipsychotic noncompliance. *Schizophr Res.* 2004;66: 51–57.
4. Birt J. Management of weight gain associated with antipsychotics. *Ann Clin Psychiatry.* 2003;15(1):49–58.
5. Centorrino F, Wurtman JJ, Duca KA, et al. Weight loss in overweight patients maintained on atypical antipsychotic agents. *Int J Obes.* 2006;30:1011–1016.
6. Barba C, Cavalli-Sforza T, Cutter J, et al. Appropriate body mass index for Asian populations and its implications for policy and intervention strategies *Lancet.* 2004;363(9403):157–163.
7. Grundy SM, Cleeman JI, Daniels SR, et al., for the American Heart Association and National Heart, Lung, and Blood Institute. Diagnosis and management of the metabolic syndrome: an American Heart Association/National Heart, Lung, and Blood Institute Scientific Statement. *Circulation.* 2005;112:2735–2752.

8. National Research Council. Committee on Diet and Health. Implications for reducing chronic disease risk. Washington, DC: National Academy Press; 1989.

9. Mendoza JA, Drewnowski A, Christakis DA. Dietary energy density is associated with obesity and the metabolic syndrome in U.S. adults. *Diabetes Care.* 2007;30(4):974–979.

10. International Diabetes Federation. The IDF consensus worldwide definition of the metabolic syndrome. http://www.idf.org/webdata/docs/IDF_Metasyndrome_definition.pdf. Accessed May 5, 2007.

11. Joslin EP. The prevention of diabetes mellitus. *JAMA.* 1921;76:79–84.

12. Haller H. Epidemiology and associated risk factors of hyperlipoproteinemia. (German). *Z Gesamte Inn Med* 1977;32(8):124–128.

13. Reaven GM. Banting lecture 1988. Role of insulin resistance in human disease. *Diabetes.* 1988;37:1595–1607.

14. McEvoy JP, Meyer JM, Goff DC, et al. Prevalence of the metabolic syndrome in patients with schizophrenia: baseline results from the clinical antipsychotic trials of intervention effectiveness (CATIE) schizophrenia trial and comparison with national estimates from NHANES III. *Schizophr Res.* 2005;80:19–32.

15. Menza M, Vreeland B, Minsky S, et al. Managing atypical antipsychotic-associated weight gain: 12 month data on a multimodal weight control program. *J Clin Psychiatry.* 2004;65(4):471–477.

16. Elvevag B, Goldberg TE. Cognitive impairment in schizophrenia is the core of the disorder. *Crit Rev Neurobiol.* 2000;14:1–21.

17. Harmatz MG, Lapuc P. Behavior modification of overeating in a psychiatric population. *J Consult Clin Psychol.* 1968;32(5):583–587.

18. Rotatori AF, Fox R, Wicks A. Weight loss with psychiatric residents in a behavioral self-control program. *Psychol Rep* 1980;46:483–486.

19. Knox JM. A study of weight reducing diets in psychiatric inpatients. *Br J Psychiatry* 1980;136:287–289.

20. Klein B, Steele RI, Simon WE, et al. Reinforcement and weight loss in schizophrenics. *Psychol Rep* 1972;30(12):581–582.

21. Sletten IW, Ognjanov V, Menendez S, et al. Weight reduction with chlorphentermine and phenmetrazine in obese psychiatric patients during chlorpromazine therapy. *Curr Ther Res Clin Exp.* 1967;9:570–575.

22. Vreeland B, Minsky S, Menza M, et al. A program for managing weight gain associated with atypical antipsychotics. *Psychiatr Serv.* 2003;54:1155–1157.

23. Ball MP, Coons VB, Buchanan RW. A program for treating olanzapine-related weight gain. *Psychiatr Serv.* 2001;52(7):967–969.

24. Littrell KH, Hilligoss NM, Kirshner CD, et al. The effects of an educational intervention on antipsychotic-induced weight gain. *J Nurs Scholar.* 2003;35(3): 237–241.

25. Brar JS, Ganguli R, Pandina G, et al. Effects of behavioral therapy on weight loss in overweight and obese patients with schizophrenia or schizoaffective disorder. *J Clin Psychiatry.* 2005;66:205–212.

26. Alvarez-Jimenez M, Gonzalez-Blanch C, Vasquez-Barquero JL, et al. Attenuation of antipsychotic-induced weight gain with early behavioral intervention in drug-naïve first episode psychosis patients: a randomized controlled trial. *J Clin Psychiatry.* 2006;67:1253–1260.

27. Kwon JS, Choi JS, Bahk WM, et al. Weight management program for treatment-emergent weight gain in olanzapine-treated patients with schizophrenia or

schizoaffective disorder: a 12-week randomized controlled clinical trial. *J Clin Psychiatry*. 2006;67:547–553.

28. O'Keefe CD, Noordsy DL, Liss TB, et al. Reversal of antipsychotic-associated weight gain. *J Clin Psychiatry*. 2003;64(8):907–912.

29. Ganguli R. Weight gain associated with antipsychotic drugs. *J Clin Psychiatry*. 1999;60(suppl 21):20–24.

30. Tuomilehto J, Lindstrom J, Eriksson JG, et al. Prevention of type 2 diabetes mellitus by changes in lifestyle among subjects with impaired glucose tolerance. *N Engl J Med*. 2001;344(18):1343–1350.

31. Pan XR, Li GW, Hu YH, et al. Effects of diet and exercise in preventing NIDDM in people with impaired glucose tolerance: the Da Qing IGT and diabetes study. *Diabetes Care*. 1997;20(4):537–544.

32. Sletten I, Mou B, Cazenave M, et al. Effects of caloric restriction on behavior and body weight during chlorpromazine therapy. *Dis Nerv Syst*. 1967;28:519–522.

33. Moore C, Crum B. Weight reduction in a chronic schizophrenic by means of operant conditioning procedures: a case study. *Behav Res Ther* 1969;7:129–131.

34. Upper D, Newton JG. A weight reduction program for schizophrenic patients on a token economy unit: two case studies. *J Behav Ther Exp Psychiatry*. 1971;2: 113–115.

35. Heimberg C, Gallacher F, Gur RC, et al. Diet and gender moderate clozapine-related weight gain. *Hum Psychopharmacol*. 1995;10:367–371.

36. Wirshing DA, Wirshing WC, Kysar L, et al. Novel antipsychotics: comparison of weight gain liabilities. *J Clin Psychiatry*. 1999;60:358–363.

37. Aquila R, Emanuel M. Interventions for weight gain in adults treated with novel antipsychotics. Primary care companion. *J Clin Psychiatry*. 2000;2:20–23.

38. Umbricht D, Flury H, Bridler R. Cognitive behavior therapy for weight gain. *Am J Psychiatry*. 2001;158:971.

39. Ganguli R, Brar J, Mullen B. Behavioral treatment for weight loss in patients with schizophrenia. Presented at the 53rd Institute of Psychiatric Services; October 10–14, 2001; Orlando FL.

40. Epstein LH. *The Stoplight Diet for Children: An Eight Week program for Parents and Children*. Boston, MA: Little Brown and Co; 1998.

41. Wolever T, Barbeau MC, Charron S, et al. Guidelines for the nutritional management of diabetes for the new millennium: a position statement by the Canadian Diabetes Association. *Can J Diabetes Care*. 1999;23(3):56–59.

42. Hortion ES. Role and management of exercise in diabetes mellitus. *Diabetes Care*. 1988;11:201–211.

43. The Diabetes Control and Complications Trial Research Group. The effect of intensive treatment of diabetes in the development and progression of long-term complications in insulin-treated diabetes mellitus. *N Engl J Med*. 1993;329:997–986.

44. U.K. Prospective Diabetes Study Group. Intensive blood glucose control with sulfonylurea or insulin compared with conventional treatment and risk of complication in patients with type 2 diabetes. *Lancet* 1998:352:837–853.

45. American Diabetes Association. National standards for diabetes self-management program and American Diabetes Association review criteria: standard 1. *Diabetes Care*. 1996;19(suppl):S114–S118.

46. Andrus M, Leggett-Frazier N, Pfeifer MA. Chronic complications of diabetes: an overview. In: Franz MJ, ed. A core curriculum for diabetes education. 5th ed. Chicago, IL: American Association of Diabetes Educators; 2003: 45–61.

47. Levey S, Adler S, Caggiula AW, et al. Effects of dietary protein restriction on the progression of advanced renal disease in the Modification of Diet in Renal Disease Study. *Am J Kidney Dis* 1996;27:652–663.
48. National Institutes of Health. Third report of the National Cholesterol Education Program (NCEP) expert panel on detection, evaluation and treatment of high blood cholesterol in adults (Adult Treatment Panel III). Executive Summary. May 2001. NIH Publication no 01-3670.
49. Escott-Stump S. Nutrition and Diagnosis-Related Care. 5th ed. Philadelphia, PA: Lippincott Williams & Wilkins; 2002: 388–389.
50. American Diabetes Association Diabetes Learning Center. http://www.diabetes.org/all-about-diabetes/chan_eng/i3/i3p4.htm. Accessed May 6, 2007.
51. Schneider SH, Morgado A. Exercise in the management of type 2 diabetes mellitus. In: Defronzo R., ed. Current therapy of diabetes mellitus. St. Louis, MO: Mosby; 1998: 90–105.
52. Fabricatore A. Behavior therapy and cognitive-behavioral therapy of obesity: is there a difference? *J Am Diet Assoc*. 2007;107:92–99.
53. McGuire MT, Wing RR, Klem ML, et al. Long-term maintenance of weight loss: do people who lose weight through various weight loss methods use different behaviors to maintain their weight? *Int J Obes Relat Metab Disord*. 1998;22:572–577.
54. Zimmerman GL, Olsen CG, Bosworth MF. A 'stages of change' approach to helping patients change behavior. *Am Fam Physician*. 2000;61(5):1409–1416.
55. International Federation for the Surgery of Obesity Selection Criteria. http://www.ifso.com/candidate.html. Accessed September 9, 2007.
56. Fabricatore AN, Crerand CE, Wadden TA, et al. How do mental health professionals evaluate candidates for bariatric surgery? Survey results. *Obes Surg*. 2006; 16(5):567–573.
57. Kalarchian M, Marcus M, Levine M, et al. Psychiatric disorders among bariatric surgery candidates: Relationship to obesity and functional health status. *Am J Psychiatry* 2007;164;328–334.
58. Hamoui N, Kingsbury S, Anthone GJ, et al. Surgical treatment of morbid obesity in schizophrenic patients. *Obes Surg*. 2004;(14)3:349–352.
59. Floris M, Lejeune J, Deberdt W. Effect of amantadine on weight gain during olanzapine treatment. *Eur Neuropsychopharmacol*. 2001;11:181–182.
60. Poyurovsky M, Isaacs I, Fuchs C, et al. Attenuation of olanzapine-induced weight gain with reboxetine in patients with schizophrenia: a double-blind, placebo-controlled study. *Am J Psychiatry*. 2003;160(2):297–302.
61. Cavazzoni P, Tanaka Y, Roychowdhury SM, et al. Nizatidine for prevention of weight gain with olanzapine: a double-blind placebo controlled trial. *Eur Neuropsychopharmacol*. 2003;13:81–85.
62. Assuncao SS, Ruschel SI, Rosa LCR, et al. Weight gain management in patients with schizophrenia during treatment with olanzapine in association with nizatidine. *Rev Bras Psiquiatr* 2006;28:270–276.
63. Poyurovsky M, Tal V, Maayan R, et al. The effect of famotidine addition on olanzapine-induced weight gain in first-episode schizophrenia patients: a double-blind placebo-controlled pilot study. *Eur Neuropsychopharmacol*. 2004;14:332–336.
64. Lin YH, Liu CY, Hsiao MC. Management of atypical antipsychotic-induced weight gain in schizophrenic patients with topiramate. *Psychiatry Clin Neurosci*. 2005; 59:613–615.

65. Baptista T, Hernandez L, Prieto LA, et al. Metformin in obesity associated with antipsychotic drug administration: a pilot study. *J Clin Psychiatry* 2001; 62(8):653–655.

66. Poyurovsky M, Pashinian A, Gil-Ad I, et al. Olanzapine-induced weight gain in patients with first-episode schizophrenia: a double-blind, placebo-controlled study of fluoxetine addition. *Am J Psychiatry.* 2002;159:1058–1060.

67. Werneke U, Taylor D, Sanders TAB. Options for pharmacological management of obesity in patients treated with atypical antipsychotics. *Int Clin Psychopharmacol.* 2002;17(4):145–160.

68. Goodall E, Oxtoby C, Richards R, et al. A clinical trial of the efficacy and acceptability of d-fenfluramine in the treatment of neuroleptic-induced obesity. *Br Psychiatry.* 1988;153:208–213.

69. Morrison J, Cottingham EM, Barton BA. Metformin for weight loss in pediatric patients taking psychotropic drugs. *Am J Psychiatry.* 2002;159(4):655–657.

70. Diabetes Prevention Program Research Group. Reduction in the incidence of type 2 diabetes with lifestyle intervention or metformin. *New Engl J Med.* 2002; 346(6):393–403.

71. Borovicka MC, Fuller MA, Konicki PE, et al. Phenylpropanolamine appears not to promote weight loss in patients with schizophrenia who have gained weight during clozapine treatment. *J Clin Psychiatry.* 2002;63:345–348.

72. Henderson DC, Copeland PM, Daley TB, et al. A double-blind, placebo-controlled trial of sibutramine for olanzapine-associated weight gain. *Am J Psychiatry.* 2005;162(5):954–962.

73. Henderson DC, Fan X, Copeland PM, et al. A double-blind, placebo-controlled trial of sibutramine for clozapine-associated weight gain. *Acta Psychiatr Scand.* 2007;115(2):101–105.

74. Dinan TG, Tobin A. Orlistat in the management of antipsychotic-induced weight gain: Two case reports. *J Serotonin Res.* 2001;7:14–15.

75. Anghelescu I, Klawe C, Benkert O. Orlistat in the treatment of psychopharmacologically induced weight gain. *J Clin Psychopharmacol* 2000;20(6):716–717.

76. National Institutes of Health. The practical guide: identification, evaluation and treatment of overweight and obesity in adults. October. 2000. NIH Publication no 00-4084. http://www.nhlbi.nih.gov/guidelines/obesity/practgde.htm. Accessed September 9, 2007.

77. National Institutes of Diabetes and Digestive and Kidney Diseases. National Institutes of Health. Obesity, physical activity and weight control glossary. http://win.niddk.nih.gov/publications/glossary/AthruL.htm. Accessed March 31, 2007,

78. ADA Nutrition Fact Sheet. Dietary Fats Clarifying and Age Old Issue. [] http://www.eatright.org. Accessed July 26, 2007.

79. Linus Pauling Institute, Oregon State University. Micronutrient Information Center. *Fiber.* Accessed March 31, 2007. http://lpi.oregonstate. edu/infocenter/phytochemicals/fiber/index.html.

CHAPTER 6

The Management of Diabetes in Patients with Mental Illness

*Vasanthi L. Narayan
and Jane E. Weinreb*

Hyperglycemia due to impaired insulin secretion or action is the hallmark of diabetes mellitus. Type 1 diabetes is classified by an absolute insulin deficiency due to beta cell destruction. Type 2 diabetes results from a slowly progressive (estimated at 5% to 10% per year) beta-cell secretory defect on the background of insulin resistance, often associated with increased visceral fat content. Affected individuals generally progress from normal glucose tolerance, to impaired glucose regulation, to overt type 2 diabetes. In addition to type 1 and type 2 diabetes, other classifications of diabetes include gestational diabetes, diabetes secondary to recognized genetic defects, diseases of the exocrine pancreas, other endocrinopathies, and drug therapies,[1] including atypical antipsychotic medications.

Preferred screening and diagnosis of diabetes is made by fasting plasma glucose measurements. A fasting plasma glucose value of 126 mg/dL or greater on more than one occasion confirms the diagnosis. Symptoms of hyperglycemia (polydipsia, polyphagia, polyuria, blurred vision, and weight loss) associated with a random plasma glucose level 200 mg/dL or greater also confirms diabetes. Although less frequently used as a screening tool, a 2-hour plasma glucose level of 200 mg/dL or greater during a 75-g oral glucose tolerance test diagnoses diabetes mellitus as well. "Prediabetes" refers to either impaired fasting glucose or impaired glucose tolerance. Impaired fasting glucose (IFG) is defined as fasting glucose values between 100 and 125 mg/dL, and impaired glucose tolerance (IGT) is defined as a 2-hour glucose value between 140 and 199 mg/dL during a 75-g oral glucose tolerance test. Both IFG and IGT suggest metabolic derangements that warrant careful monitoring to prevent progression to overt diabetes mellitus.[1]

Given the growing prevalence of diabetes mellitus, criteria for population-based screening are evolving. The United States Preventive Task Force does not recommend routine diabetes screening, because universal screening has not been shown to be of benefit. However, given the increased risk of cardio-vascular disease in patients with diabetes, the task force recommends screening adults with hypertension and dyslipidemia for diabetes.[2,3] In contrast, the American Diabetes Association (ADA) notes that many patients with diabetes present with complications and suggests that these complications could be prevented with earlier diagnosis and glycemic control.[1]

Current recommendations by the ADA for screening in the general population include obtaining fasting plasma glucose in patients older than 45 years of age, especially in those with a body mass index (BMI) greater than 25; if BMI values are normal, the test can be repeated in 3 years. Screening of younger patients is recommended if the BMI is greater 25 and there is at least one additional risk factor. These include physical inactivity, a positive family history of diabetes mellitus (first-degree relative), being a member of a high-risk ethnic group (African American, Latino, Native American, Asian American, or Pacific Islander), delivery of an infant who weighed greater than 9 lb, the presence of gestational diabetes, a concomitant diagnosis of hypertension, vascular disease, valvular heart disease or dyslipidemia (specifically high-density lipoprotein [HDL] cholesterol less than 35 mg/dL and/or triglyc-erides greater than 250 mg/dL), or signs of insulin resistance, including polycystic ovarian syndrome or acanthosis nigricans. Yearly evaluation is rec-ommended for individuals with IFG or IGT on previous testing.[1] Some data suggest that patients with schizophrenia and schizoaffective disorders are at increased risk for diabetes and hence warrant screening along with these other high-risk groups.[4,5]

Once diabetes is diagnosed, other clinical and laboratory data can provide guidance on risk stratification and treatment strategies. Mortality in diabetes is increased due to cardiovascular disease; thus aggressive cardiovascular disease risk factor modification is appropriate. Important laboratory parameters to evaluate include glycosylated hemoglobin (A_{1c}) as an indicator of chronic glycemic control, blood pressure, lipid profile (low-density lipoprotein [LDL] cholesterol, HDL cholesterol, triglycerides, and total cholesterol), liver func-tion tests, and evaluation of renal function with serum creatinine and urinaly-sis to evaluate for microalbuminuria, frank proteinuria, or glycosuria. Family history of diabetes or early cardiac disease needs to be ascertained. Patients should be questioned for any symptoms of cardiac, renal, or vascular disease. Other conditions that may be causing or contributing to hyperglycemia (i.e., either endogenous or exogenous hypercortisolism, acromegaly, thyroid dis-ease, or other endocrinopathy) should be considered.[1]

Diabetes treatment goals are largely derived from landmark trials. The Diabetes Control and Complication Trial (DCCT) studied intensive versus conventional glycemic control (A_{1c} of 7.2% vs. 9%) in type 1 diabetes. The risk of development or progression of microvascular complications was decreased by 50% to 75% in those patients who achieved intensive control.[6] Follow-up data from the DCCT in the Epidemiology of Diabetes Interventions and

Complications (EDIC) trial suggested a reduction in macrovascular complications as well.[7] However, this level of control was also associated with a three-fold increase in the risk of severe hypoglycemia.[6] The United Kingdom Prospective Diabetes Study (UKPDS) compared intensive versus conventional glycemic control (A_{1c} 7% vs. 7.9%) in more than 4,000 newly diagnosed type 2 diabetics. Results revealed that intensive control resulted in a 25% reduction in development of microvascular complications, translating into approximately a 35% reduction for each 1% decrease in A_{1c}. Furthermore, a 16% reduction in the combined fatal and nonfatal myocardial infarction and sudden death occurred in the intensive control group.[8] Additionally, aggressive control of hypertension in patients with type 2 diabetes in UKPDS significantly reduced strokes, diabetes-related deaths, heart failure, and vision loss.[9]

Based on these trials, therapeutic goals of diabetes care are aimed at lowering blood glucose levels to near normal with avoidance of hypoglycemic episodes. Treatment is mandated to reduce the risk of acute decompensation, including diabetic ketoacidosis or hyperglycemic crisis; to alleviate symptoms of hyperglycemia; and to reduce the risk of development and/or progression of microvascular and macrovascular complications, including risks of cardiovascular disease.

Glycemic targets suggested by the ADA include preprandial plasma glucose values between 90 and 130 mg/dL (80–120 mg/dL capillary whole blood glucose), and 2-hour postprandial plasma glucose values of less than 180 mg/dl (<170 mg/dL capillary whole blood glucose). The ADA recommends A_{1c} levels of less than 7.0% (or <1% above normal values). Expert opinion suggests that less intensive goals are appropriate in patients with severe or frequent hypoglycemia, the very young, the very old, or those with modest or advanced microvascular disease or other major comorbidities.[1] Some individuals with severe psychiatric illness may similarly benefit from modified glycemic goals.

In addition to glycemic goals, several nonglycemic goals are also recommended for people with diabetes, specifically aimed to modify other cardiovascular risk factors. These include blood pressure control, the use of aspirin, lipid control and eliminating tobacco use. Hypertension contributes to the development and progression of many diabetic complications, including cardiovascular and cerebrovascular disease, retinopathy, and nephropathy. Control of hypertension has clearly been shown to decrease the rate of these complications. The goal blood pressure in patients with diabetes is less than 130/80 mm Hg. For blood pressures between 130–139/80–89 mm Hg, lifestyle changes may be attempted for 3 months, after which drug treatment should be initiated for continued elevation above target values. For blood pressure greater than 140 mm Hg systolic or 90 mm Hg diastolic, patients should begin pharmacological therapy along with lifestyle changes.[1] Initial drug treatment should be with an angiotensin-converting enzyme (ACE) inhibitor or angiotensin receptor blocker (ARB), both of which offer renal protection (especially if patient has microalbuminuria), unless contraindicated.[10,11] Other appropriate antihypertensive choices include diuretics, beta-blockers (especially in patients with prior diagnosis of coronary artery disease), or nondihydropyridine calcium channel blockers.

Diabetes is considered a coronary artery disease equivalent by the National Cholesterol Education Panel (NCEP) III.[12] Aspirin therapy is considered a routine part of secondary prevention in people with diabetes and a history of cardiovascular disease, and it is also recommended as part of primary prevention for cardiovascular disease in all patients with diabetes older than 40 years of age; additionally treatment with 75 to 325 mg/day of aspirin should be considered in patients 30 to 40 years of age with one additional cardiovascular risk factor.[1,13] The primary goal of lipid therapy is LDL lowering, because this has been independently associated with a reduction of cardiovascular events. The primary LDL goal for diabetics is less than 100 mg/dL; additionally, for all people older than 40 years of age with diabetes, statin therapy is recommended to lower the LDL by 30% to 40%, regardless of baseline levels.[14] In diabetic patients with known coronary artery disease, goals for LDL levels may be even lower, at less than 70 mg/dL. Secondary treatment goals include a non-HDL cholesterol (i.e., total cholesterol minus HDL) less than 130 mg/dL, and an increase in HDL to >40 mg/dL in men and >50 mg/dL in women. Lowering triglycerides to levels less than 150 mg/dL also confers cardiovascular benefit.[1,14] However, hyperglycemia and hypertriglyceridemia are intricately linked, likely through elevations of free fatty acids. Free fatty acids are potent inhibitors of insulin action and transport, and act to disrupt glucose transport into skeletal muscle. Thus, triglyceride goals are often difficult to attain in uncontrolled diabetes. Second-generation antipsychotics may also adversely affect triglyceride levels.[15-17]

Treatment for all dyslipidemias must involve lifestyle changes, including a low cholesterol and low fat diet, weight loss, and exercise. Pharmacotherapy for LDL reduction includes statins, resins, high-dose niacin preparations, and ezetimibe. Hypertriglyceridemia can be treated with fibrates, omega-3 fatty acids, abstinence from alcohol, weight loss, and improved glycemic control. Unfortunately, low HDL lacks many effective therapies; fibrates and niacin derivatives offer some benefit, as do exercise, weight loss, and smoking cessation. Moderate consumption of alcohol to raise HDL remains controversial.[1]

Tobacco use is associated with an increased risk of morbidity and mortality due to development and progression of microvascular and macrovascular complications in diabetic patients. Counseling on smoking cessation should be included as a routine part of diabetes care, and has been shown effective in decreasing tobacco consumption.[1] Thus, smoking cessation should be addressed as part of every physician encounter. For complex reasons, patients with mental illness, specifically schizophrenia, are more likely to be nicotine-dependent as well as consume more nicotine products, further contributing to cardiovascular risk.[18,19] Counseling, especially if individualized to the motivated patient, can be helpful; however, given the complexity of nicotine dependence in this population, counseling may prove to be less effective in long-term smoking cessation.[20]

In summary, all patients with diabetes should have fasting plasma glucose, A_{1c}, lipid levels, and blood pressure assessed at baseline and every 3 months during management. In patients who are well-controlled and on a stable drug regimen, monitoring can continue at 6-month intervals. Smoking cessation should be addressed at each physician encounter. A recent consensus conference recommended a specific protocol to monitor patients being treated with second-generation antipsychotics. This protocol included measurement and follow-up of recommended parameters (weight, waist circumference, blood pressure, fasting plasma glucose, fasting lipid profile) at regular intervals to permit earlier diagnosis and therapeutic modification if severe metabolic derangements were observed.[21] In patients with known diabetes mellitus who are to be started on antipsychotic therapy, history regarding age and circumstances of diagnosis (i.e., acute hospitalization or routine laboratory work), drug therapies used in the past and currently, and hyperglycemic or hypoglycemic emergencies encountered, help provide guidance in continued management.

All patients with diabetes should be referred to comprehensive diabetes education programs, including instruction in home glucose monitoring, intensive medical nutrition therapy, exercise programs, and insulin administration as necessary.[1] Individual patient sessions with a nutritionist and certified diabetes educator may also prove useful for reinforcement of educational guidelines. Family members and caregivers should be encouraged to attend education sessions and physician visits to help facilitate patient adherence to treatment plans.

Diabetic patients, including those with psychiatric comorbidity, should have routine follow-up care and management of cardiovascular risk factors, preferably by an internist. For patients with poorly controlled diabetes ($A_{1c} > 8\%$) at baseline, early referral to a diabetologist or endocrinologist should be encouraged. Additionally, referrals are necessary for patients prescribed second-generation antipsychotics if their diabetes is newly diagnosed with initial screening, or if glycemic control worsens (rise in $A_{1c} >1\%$ or to $>8\%$) with initiation of treatment.

Diagnostic cardiac stress testing should be performed in any patient with symptoms of typical or atypical chest pain, or with a resting electrocardiogram suggestive of ischemia or infarct. Risk stratification by exercise or nuclear stress testing is recommended in any patient with a history of cardiovascular, peripheral vascular, or carotid vascular disease, or in any patient older than 35 years of age with a history of a sedentary lifestyle who is planning to initiate a vigorous exercise program.[1] If a patient has any history or symptoms of cardiac or vascular disease, referrals to cardiology or vascular surgery should be made by the primary provider.

Diabetic nephropathy occurs in 20% to 40% of patients with diabetes and is the leading cause of end-stage renal disease in the United States. Persistent microalbuminuria (defined as 30 to 299 mg albumin/day collected over 24 hours), or spot urine albumin to creatinine ratio of 0.03 to 0.3 verified by repeat testing, defines the earliest stage of diabetic nephropathy.[1] The presence of microalbuminuria and overt nephropathy serves as an independent predictor or marker of cardiovascular disease.[22] Serum creatinine should be measured at least annually in all diabetic patients with more frequent testing recommended during initiation of treatment with possibly nephrotoxic medications. ACE inhibitors have been shown to be effective in slowing the progression of renal disease in people with type 1 and in people with type 2 diabetes and hypertension with evidence of microalbuminuria.[10] For patients with serum creatinine levels greater than 1.5 mg/dL with hypertension and evidence of macroalbuminuria, ARBs are recommended.[11] As discussed, blood pressure control needs to be optimized to reduce the risk and slow progression of intrinsic diabetic renal disease. In patients with overt nephropathy, protein restriction (0.8 g/kg/day) should be initiated. If evaluation indicates signs of progressive renal disease (glomerular filtrate rate <60 mL/min), or if hypertension or potassium balance is difficult to manage, a nephrologist should be involved in the care of the patient.

Diabetic retinopathy is the most frequent cause of blindness among adults 20 to 74 years of age and is often worsened by coexisting hypertension. To slow the risk and progression of retinopathy, early referral to ophthalmology for dilated funduscopic examination is necessary. For patients with type 1 diabetes, referral to ophthalmology is recommended within 3 to 5 years of initial diagnosis. However, referrals should be made earlier for patients with type 2 diabetes because the majority have longer-standing disease at the time of diagnosis. For patients with high-risk characteristics or macular edema, laser treatment can be considered by the eye specialist. If patients have a normal examination, follow-up dilated retinal examination can be deferred to every 2 years. In contrast, in the setting of high-risk characteristics, including nonproliferative or proliferative disease, follow-up should be at least annually.[1] Optimization of glycemic and blood pressure control can help abate the progression of retinopathy.[6]

Peripheral neuropathies associated with diabetes can cause pain, decreased sensation, or weakness in the extremities. The primary care provider should provide comprehensive foot care education and screening for distal symmetric polyneuropathy at the time of diagnosis and annually thereafter in all patients with type 2 diabetes. Patients with neuropathy should have a visual inspection of their feet at each physician visit. Screening should be performed with at least two modalities (i.e., 10-g monofilament and a tuning fork) for greater sensitivity. The loss of two sensory modalities predicts increased risk of foot ulcers. A multidisciplinary approach including early referral to podiatry is recommended for patients with a high risk examination or foot ulcers. High-risk feet include those with decreased protective sensation, deformities, nail pathology, peripheral vascular disease, or a history of prior ulcers. Well-fitted walking shoes are recommended for patients with neuropathy or evidence of increased plantar pressure.[1] The most widely used medical treatments for symptoms of diabetic neuropathy include gabapentin and tricyclic antidepressants. These agents should be used cautiously and with appropriate psychiatric consultation in patients with coexisting psychiatric disease.[23]

The risks of progressive neuropathy and amputation are increased significantly in patients who have had diabetes for more than 10 years, in male patients, and in those with poor glycemic control; risks are also increased in those with other diabetic complications, including cardiovascular, retinal, or renal complications. Autonomic neuropathies can affect gastrointestinal, genitourinary, and cardiovascular function. Clinical signs of autonomic neuropathies include resting tachycardia, orthostasis, gastroparesis, or recurrent urinary tract infections. Tight glycemic control can diminish the onset and progression of peripheral and autonomic neuropathies.[1,6,7]

Treatment strategies for hyperglycemia, hyperinsulinemia, prediabetes, or frank diabetes continue to evolve with the results of recent data, newer formulations of oral agents and insulin, and the development of alternative therapeutic targets. If glycemic dysregulation is associated with a particular antipsychotic therapy and diagnosed early, glycemic management can be addressed, if feasible, by changing antipsychotic therapy. Specifically, clozapine and olanzapine have shown the highest propensity for weight gain, diabetes risk, and worsening lipid profile; aripiprazole and ziprasidone have shown the least. Quetiapine and risperidone have both been associated with weight gain, although the risk of diabetes and dyslipidemia is thought to be less than that of clozapine or olanzapine.[21] Thus, in addition to psychiatric benefit offered, metabolic risk factors may need to be considered when prescribing antipsychotic therapy.

Intensive lifestyle modification with the goal of weight loss, including dietary counseling and exercise, should be included as a fundamental component of any effective management program for patients with diabetes, prediabetes, or other cardiovascular risk factors.[1] Positive results from several randomized controlled trials using lifestyle intervention have become available in recent years. Specifically, the U.S. Diabetes Prevention Program (DPP)[24,25] and the Finnish Diabetes Prevention Study (DPS)[26] found that reduction in body weight achieved through an intensive diet and exercise program reduced the incidence of type 2 diabetes in adults with IGT. The DPS participants who remained free of diabetes at the close of the study were followed for an additional 3 years after the discontinuation of individual counseling. Extended follow-up data revealed that the incidence of diabetes remained reduced with maintenance of beneficial lifestyle changes.[26,27] Although often not sustainable, these studies suggest both short and long-term benefit of weight loss and lifestyle modification in diabetes prevention.

The treatment of diabetes mellitus continues to evolve with the introduction of new drug classes (Table 6.1) and new formulations of insulin (Table 6.2). The choice of a specific antihyperglycemic agent is based on effectiveness in lowering glucose, as well as safety profile, tolerability, and expense; therapy varies based on baseline level of glycemic control and beta

Table 6.1   Oral hypoglycemic agents

Drug class and names	Mechanism of action	Dosing	Advantages	Efficacy	Side effects	Uses
Sulfonylureas (Glyburide, Glipizide, Glimepiride, Chlorpropamide)	Binds to specific receptors on beta cell to stimulate insulin release	Glyburide 2.5–20 mg/d; Glipizide 5–40 mg/d; Glimepiride 1–8 mg/d; Chlorpropamide 100–500 mg/d	Inexpensive, long history of safety	↓ A_{1c} by 1.5%–2%; ↓ FBG by 60 mg/dL	Hypoglycemia, weight gain; caution in elderly or in renal diseases	Consider use in lean type 2 diabetics with beta cell function; use with other OHA or HS insulin
Meglitinides (Repaglinide, Nateglinide)	Binds to non-SU receptors on beta cell to stimulate insulin release	Repaglinide 0.5–4 mg premeal; Nateglinide 60–120 mg premeal	Rapid onset and offset, dietary variability permitted, hepatic metabolism	Repaglinide similar to SU; nateglinide ↓ A_{1c} 0.5%–0.8%	Hypoglycemia, caution in liver disease	Patients with erratic meal patterns, renal disease; use with other OHA or bedtime insulin
Biguanides (Metformin)	↓ gluconeogenesis, ↑ peripheral insulin sensitivity, anorectic effect	Initiate 500–850 mg premeal, increase to maximum 2000 mg/d	Limited hypoglycemia, weight-neutral	Similar to SU	GI discomfort, avoid use in patients with renal disease, caution lactic acidosis	First-line OHA especially obese; use with other OHAs and/or insulin

Drug class	Mechanism	Dosing	Advantages	Efficacy	Disadvantages	Comments
Alpha-glucosidase inhibitors (Acarbose, Miglitol)	Delays carbohydrate absorption by inhibiting intestinal glucosidases	Initiate 25 mg premeal, increase to maximum of 100 mg three times daily	↓ Postprandial insulin levels, limited hypoglycemia	↓ A_{1c} by 0.5%–1.0%, ↓ postprandial BG by 50–60 mg/dL	GI discomfort, avoid use in patients with liver disease; caution hypoglycemia with other OHA	Consider in patients with normal FBG but high postprandial BG; use with other OHA and/or insulin
Thiazolidinediones (Rosiglitazone, Pioglitazone)	PPARγ receptor agonists ↑ peripheral insulin sensitivity at muscle and fat	Rosiglitazone 2–8 mg/d; Pioglitazone 15–45 mg/d	Limited hypoglycemia, favorable lipid profile	↓ A_{1c} by 0.5%–1.0%, ↓ FBG by 15–60 mg/dL	Weight gain (with insulin), fluid retention, edema, anemia, caution in liver disease, congestive heart failure	Use in obese patients with type 2 diabetes mellitus; use with other OHA and/or insulin
DPP-IV inhibitors (Sitagliptin)	Inhibition of dipeptidylpeptidase IV → ↑ circulating GIP and GLP-1	100 mg/d; adjust dose in renal disease	Once daily dosing, limited hypoglycemia, weight-neutral, few side effects	↓ A_{1c} by 0.5%–1.0%, ↓ FBG and postprandial BG	Limited	Use as monotherapy or in combination with biguanides and/or thiazolidinediones; limited data of use with insulin

FBG = fasting blood glucose, SU = sulfonylureas, OHA = oral hypoglycemic agents, GI = gastrointestinal; BG = blood glucose.

Table **6.2** Insulin regimens						
Insulin preparation	Onset of action (h)	Peak action (h)	Duration of action (h)	Advantages	Disadvantages	Uses
Regular (R) (soluble, unmodified, clear)	0.5–1	2–4	6–8	Inexpensive, long track record	Need to take 30–60 minutes prior to meal	Premeal SQ; IV/IM[a] for management of crisis
Insulin analogues (Lispro, Aspart, or Glulisine)	0.25–0.5	1–2	3–6	Can use at meals, less variable onset and duration, intensive blood glucose (postprandial) control, less hypoglycemia	More expensive, may have period of relative hypoinsulinization between injections, more rapid onset of DKA with insulin pump failure	Premeal SQ, IV, pumps
NPH insulin (N) (cloudy, modified)	1–4 (average 2)	8–10	12–20	Inexpensive; can mix with R (no change in insulin kinetics)	Not truly flat; peaks in late PM if used in AM and at 2:00–3:00 AM if used predinner	Basal insulinization at bedtime, bid, qid with tube feeds
70/30 insulin (70% N, 30% R)	0.5–1	Dual	12–20	Premixed, helpful in elderly, blind	Limited flexibility, often preventing tight control	Insulinization for those unable to mix insulin
50/50 Insulin (50% N, 50% R)	0.5–1	Dual	12–20	Premixed, helpful in elderly, blind	Limited flexibility, often preventing tight control	Insulinization for those unable to mix insulin

| Glargine | 1.5 | None | 20.5–23 | Provides flat basal insulinization | More expensive, cannot be mixed with other insulins, requires extra injection, more injection site pain | Basal insulinization, given every day; can be part of basal/prandial insulin regimen or with oral hypoglycemic agents |
| Detemir | | ? None | Variable, dose-related | Provides approximately flat basal insulinization | More expensive, need to split dose twice-daily if dose <0.5 U/kg body weight | Daily or twice daily as basal insulinization |

[a]When used intravenously, onset ~ immediate, with circulating half-life of 6 minutes, peak glucose lowering in 20–30 minutes, and full effect dissipated in 2–3 hours. When used intramuscularly, blood glucose nadir reached in 60–90 minutes, with some persistent activity for 3–4 hours.
DKA = diabetic ketoacidosis.

cell secretory capacity. Because type 2 diabetes is a progressive disease, addition of medications over time is almost always necessary. Well-known classes of oral agents include sulfonylureas, meglitinides, biguanides, α-glucosidase inhibitors, and thiazolidinediones.[28]

The sulfonylureas (glipizide, glyburide) act as insulin secretagogues and stimulate pancreatic beta cells to release insulin, reducing A_{1c} by 1.5% to 2%. The major adverse effect of the sulfonylurea class is hypoglycemia, often more frequent and severe in elderly patients or in those with renal dysfunction. Meglitinides (repaglinide, nateglinide) act similarly to sulfonylureas but bind to a different site on the sulfonylurea receptor. These agents are administered just prior to meals to maximize endogenous insulin secretory capacity in the presence of a carbohydrate load. Meglitinides are metabolized by the liver and are generally preferred in patients with renal insufficiency. This class has a rapid onset and offset of action and therefore is also preferred in patients who do not eat consistent meals. Both sulfonylureas and meglitinides are dependent on endogenous capacity to secrete insulin and therefore are not indicated in those patients without beta cell function. Unfortunately, weight gain is common with these agents. The impact of sulfonylureas as a class on cardiovascular mortality has not been substantiated.[29]

Biguanides (metformin) are generally considered first-line therapy for nearly all patients with type 2 diabetes without contraindication (i.e., decompensated heart failure, renal failure). These agents act by inhibition of hepatic gluconeogenesis, lowering fasting glucose levels and improving insulin sensitivity. Typically, metformin monotherapy reduces A_{1c} by 1.5%. Therapy is usually not associated with hypoglycemia or weight gain, and the drug promotes modest weight loss in some patients. Side effects include mild gastrointestinal symptoms, or rarely, severe lactic acidosis. Effects of metformin monotherapy on cardiovascular outcomes are currently being investigated, though limited data from the UKPDS suggests some cardiovascular benefit in obese patients with type 2 diabetes.[30]

The α-glucosidase inhibitors reduce the rate of absorption of polysaccharides in the small intestine and thereby lower postprandial glucose levels without significant hypoglycemia; however, these agents are less effective than metformin or sulfonylureas. Given the unpleasant side effect profile of increased flatulence and gastrointestinal discomfort, discontinuation rates are high. Potential benefits of α-glucosidase inhibitors in cardiovascular disease outcomes need to be further investigated.[31,32]

Thiazolidinediones (rosiglitazone, pioglitazone) act as agonists of the peroxisome proliferator-activator receptor gamma and improve insulin sensitivity at the tissue level. These agents are contraindicated in patients with heart failure and can worsen peripheral edema. Unfortunately, a common side effect of the glitazone class of agents is weight gain. This effect is thought to be due in part to redistribution of fat from visceral stores resulting in subcutaneous adiposity; these changes may be further augmented by the weight gain known to accompany several antipsychotic agents. The thiazolidinediones may have a beneficial effect on atherogenic lipid profiles, but recent studies suggest this may not result in impaired cardiovascular outcomes.[33] Additionally, these drugs appear to decrease appendicular bone mass with associated increased risk of fractures.[34] Recently, the Diabetes REduction Assessment with Ramipril and rosiglitazone Medication (DREAM) study suggested benefit of rosiglitazone in preventing the progression of prediabetes to frank diabetes mellitus; however, drug therapy for diabetes prevention is not yet standard practice.[35]

Recently introduced into the antidiabetes market are agents that help mimic the incretin effect. The incretins, specifically GIP and GLP-1, are gut hormones released postprandially from K-and L-cells of the small intestine and colon. These peptides stimulate the secretion of insulin through enhancement of beta cell responsiveness. They also inhibit glucagon release, delay gastric emptying, and enhance satiety. In animal models, GLP-1 may stimulate beta cell proliferation and insulin biosynthesis, as well as inhibit apoptosis of human islets.[36] Endogenous GLP-1 is rapidly degraded by the enzyme dipeptidyl peptidase–IV (DPP-IV). Therefore, inhibition of DPP-IV increases active endogenous portal GLP-1. Longer acting synthetic GLP-1 analogues and DPP-IV inhibitors have recently been introduced; many other GLP-1 receptor agonists are under development. Monotherapy with GLP-1 analogues or DPP-IV inhibitors appears to lower A_{1c} by 0.5% to 1.0%, mainly through reduction of postprandial glucose values without significant hypoglycemia. A single GLP-1 analogue, exenatide, is currently available and is administered as twice-daily subcutaneous injections; this agent may also promote significant weight loss, although gastrointestinal side effects are common. The DPP-IV inhibitors (sitagliptin) are oral agents taken once daily; these drugs are weight-neutral and have a more favorable side-effect profile, which may facilitate adherence.[28]

Another recent development in diabetes management includes amylin analogues. Amylin is a peptide that is with insulin from beta cells when stimulated by carbohydrate intake; people with insulin-deficient diabetes also lack amylin. Actions of amylin include inhibition of both gastric emptying and glucagon secretion in a glucose-dependent fashion; some studies have shown that inhibition of food intake occurs, resulting in weight loss in the long term. However, similar to the GLP-1 analogue exenatide, synthetic amylin (pramlintide) may cause mild to moderate nausea, which may be responsible for weight loss. Additionally, pramlintide use has been associated with severe hypoglycemia. Pramlintide can be used in insulin-deficient patients with type 1 and type 2 diabetes, and is given as a premeal injection in conjunction with insulin therapy. Widespread use of amylin analogues in diabetes treatment has been limited.[28]

Insulin therapy has been the mainstay of diabetes medications and remains the most effective treatment. When used in adequate doses to overcome insulin resistance in type 2 diabetes, insulin can decrease any level of elevated A_{1c} into the target range. Until recently, available regimens consisted of multiple daily injections of intermediate-acting (12 to 20 hours) neutral protamine Hagedorn (NPH) insulin with short-acting (6 to 10 hours)

Regular (R) insulin or premixed 70/30 formulations. As more information became available about the true peaks and plateaus of action of these insulins, formulations were created to mimic physiological basal and prandial insulin release.

Basal insulin therapy (specifically, insulin glargine and detemir) has been developed to have a more prolonged duration, and thereby to decrease daily glycemic variability. These longer acting basal formulations were also shown to have less weight gain and less hypoglycemia than conventional insulin therapy. Prandial insulin therapy now consists of the rapid-acting insulin analogues aspart, glulisine, and lispro. Because these insulins are only to be taken in the presence of food, hypoglycemic episodes resulting from inconsistent meal patterns are reduced and post prandial glycemic control is improved.[28]

Deficits in current insulin regimens include physician resistance to initiate therapy, patient fear of injections, variable rates of insulin absorption and variable duration of action, hypoglycemia from tight control or from inconsistent meal patterns, weight gain, and lack of preservation of beta cell function. Conservative initiation of insulin therapy is usually started with bedtime NPH (usually 10 units) with titration to goal fasting sugars between 90 and 130 mg/dL. Alternatively, insulin therapy can be initiated on a weight basis starting with approximately 0.3 units/kg divided into basal and mealtime components with titration as indicated. Endocrinology consultants are readily available to assist with insulin dosing for patients who will be initiated on exogenous insulin therapy.

Guidelines for initiation of diabetes therapy have recently been published.[28] The algorithm recommends lifestyle intervention with metformin as first-line therapy unless contraindicated, with titration to maximal effective dose over 1 to 2 months. If hyperglycemia persists, another agent should be added within 2 to 3 months of treatment initiation, or at any time when A_{1c} is not at goal. Second-line treatments include sulfonylureas, glitazones, or basal insulin, with insulin preferred if A_{1c} is greater than 8.5%. If A_{1c} goals are still not achieved, but A_{1c} is less than 8%, a third oral agent can be considered, although it is less likely to be effective. If A_{1c} is greater than 8%, insulin therapy should be initiated or intensified (i.e., prandial component added). As additional agents are added, mechanistic synergy of particular combinations should be considered. For instance, once prandial insulin coverage is added, insulin secretagogues can be discontinued. Insulin therapy (with lifestyle modification) is the first-line treatment if the A_{1c} is greater than 10%, fasting blood glucose levels are greater than 250 mg/dL, or random glucoses are greater than 300 mg/dL, because doses can be titrated rapidly to achieve glucose targets. Once glucose toxicity, and potentially beta cell toxicity, is reversed, oral agents may be considered. Finally, as discussed, several new agents have entered the market and may be effective treatment options, especially for earlier stages of disease.

The development of diabetes associated with initiation of antipsychotic agents adds many challenges to the health burden of patients with coexisting mental illness who may lack the capacity to follow antidiabetic treatments. Cornerstones of diabetes management include comprehensive education with patient involvement in self-management; lifestyle interventions, including dietary modifications, exercise, and smoking cessation; home monitoring of blood glucose values to evaluate treatment regimens; and adherence to likely multiple medications and many physician encounters.

Medical nutrition therapy is a critical part of diabetes care. Patients are encouraged to monitor dietary intake, to learn to manage carbohydrate intake, to eat regular meals with consistent carbohydrate counts, and to avoid frequent (and detrimental) snacking. Patients need to modify consumption of high-fat foods, as well as foods and beverages rich in sugar, including regular soda, juice, candy and snack foods. Many antipsychotic medications contribute to irregular and more frequent consumption of food, likely through interaction of atypical antipsychotic medications with dopamine, serotonin, and histamine neuronal receptors. More specifically, the blockade of 5-HT2 receptors may lead to appetite dysregulation.[37] These patterns can result in consumption of foods that both adversely affect glycemic control and result in weight gain which further complicates management of diabetes. Psychiatric patients with diabetes who are institutionalized or living at board-and-care facilities may lack dietary choices; as a result, food consumption may be inconsistent, erratic, or inappropriate for optimal glycemic control. Finally, for those patients who require insulin therapy, ideal prandial coverage is determined by matching insulin dosing to carbohydrate consumption. Mastering prandial coverage requires the patient to perform calculations that may be difficult due to coexisting psychiatric illness.

Exercise is an important part of diabetes management, not only for weight management, but also to aid in improving insulin sensitivity. Recommendations include moderate daily exercise for at least 30 to 45 minutes most days of the week.[1] Even for the general population, setting aside the time and expending the energy to exercise requires considerable motivation. For those with psychiatric disease, this challenge may be even greater and can be thwarted by the manifestations of coexisting illness.

Smoking is an independent cardiovascular risk factor and often contributes to the development and progression of both microvascular and macrovascular diabetic complications.[1] However, smoking is often considered an integral component of psychiatric illness, especially schizophrenia.[18] Given the multiple components of diabetes care that affect the routine and lifestyle of patients with this disease, mandating smoking cessation is necessary though challenging.[20]

Self-monitoring of blood glucose is an important element in adjusting or adding new interventions, particularly during titration of insulin doses. The need for and number of required measurements is not clear and often depends on medications prescribed.[1] Ideally, various combinations of fasting, premeal, bedtime, and 2-hour postprandial glucose readings will be monitored while insulin therapy is being adjusted. Even in the nonpsychiatric population, patients often do not comply with such frequent glucose monitoring. Obtaining these values in patients with psychiatric illness is often complicated unless the patient is hospitalized.

In addition to glycemic goals, nonglycemic treatment goals of blood pressure control, lipid management, and initiation of aspirin therapy are often necessary. For many patients, the diagnosis of diabetes results in multidrug therapy. For patients with mental illness who are likely to already be on multiple medications, the addition of several new agents can be difficult. Several studies have suggested that medication adherence in patients with psychiatric illness is poor at baseline,[38] and may worsen when an increasing number of medications are prescribed. Furthermore, the diagnosis of diabetes often necessitates multidisciplinary involvement in patient care, including diabetes educators, nutritionists, endocrinologists, ophthalmologists, podiatrists, and potentially subspecialists, such as nephrologists or cardiologists. For patients with mental illness, the addition of many new providers and physician visits may be perceived as overwhelming, and adherence may be adversely affected.

Finally, because of the very nature of psychiatric illness, there may be difficulty in recognizing the signs and symptoms of the extremes of glycemic control. The neuropsychiatric manifestations of untreated hyperglycemia and hypoglycemia can be easily confused with deteriorating or unstable mental illness. Astute awareness is required to recognize and treat glycemic deterioration rapidly prior to assuming an underlying psychiatric cause. Additionally, in the setting of decompensated mental illness, medication and dietary noncompliance may be more likely. Thus, metabolic deterioration should be evaluated during psychiatric decompensation.

In practice, patients likely to be treated with second-generation antipsychotics include those with schizophrenia spectrum disorders, bipolar disorder, dementia, psychotic depression, autism, and other developmental disorders. Even though some of these medications may be associated an increased risk of metabolic side effects, the psychiatric benefit to a specific patient could outweigh potential risks. Therefore, as a medical community, clinicians must be cognizant of these associations and carefully monitor patients for the development of hyperglycemia and related complications. Providers from many disciplines and specialties must work collaboratively to provide effective care to manage this medically complicated disease process that afflicts challenging patient population.

References

1. American Diabetes Association. Standards of Medical Care in Diabetes—2007. *Diabetes Care*. 2007;30(1):S4–41.
2. United States Preventive Services Task Force. Screening for type 2 diabetes mellitus in adults: recommendations and rationale. *Ann Intern Med*. 2003;138(3):212–214.

3. Hoerger TJ, Harris R, Hicks KA, et al. Screening for type 2 diabetes mellitus: a cost-effectiveness analysis. *Ann Intern Med*. 2004;140(9):689–700.

4. Cohen D, Stolk RP, Grobbee DE, et al. Hyperglycemia and diabetes in patients with schizophrenia or schizoaffective disorders. *Diabetes Care*. 2006;29(4): 786–791.

5. Lean ME, Pajonk FG. Patients on atypical antipsychotic drugs—another high-risk group for type 2 diabetes. *Diabetes Care*. 2003;26(5):1597–1605.

6. The Diabetes Control and Complications Research Group. The effect of intensive diabetes treatment on the development and progression of long-term complications in insulin-dependent diabetes mellitus: the Diabetes Control and Complications Trial. *New Engl J Med*. 1993;329:977–986.

7. The Diabetes Control and Complications Trial/Epidemiology of Diabetes Intervention Complications (DCCT/EDIC) Study Group. Intensive diabetes treatment and cardiovascular disease in patients with type 1 diabetes. *New Engl J Med*. 2005;353(25):2643–2653.

8. UK Prospective Diabetes Study (UKPDS) Group. Intensive blood-glucose control with sulfonylureas or insulin compared with conventional treatment and risk of complications in patients with type 2 diabetes (UKPDS 33). *Lancet*. 1998;352: 837–853.

9. UK Prospective Diabetes Study (UKPDS) Group. Tight blood pressure control and risk of macrovascular and microvascular complications in type 2 diabetes (UKPDS 38). *BMJ*. 1998;317:703–713.

10. The Heart Outcomes Prevention Evaluation (HOPE) Study Investigators. Effect of an angiotensin converting enzyme inhibitor, ramipril, on cardiovascular events in high risk patients. *New Engl J Med*. 2000;342(3):145–153.

11. Lewis EJ, Hunsicker LG, Clarke WR, et al. Renoprotective effects of the angiotensin-receptor antagonist irbesartan in patients with nephropathy due to type 2 diabetes. *New Engl J Med*. 2001;345(12):851–860.

12. Grundy SM, Cleemen J, Mers CN, et al. Implications of recent clinical trials for the National Cholesterol Education Program Adult Treatment Panel III guidelines. *Circulation*. 2004;110:227–239.

13. American Diabetes Association. Aspirin therapy in diabetes. *Diabetes Care*. 2004: 27:S72–73.

14. Collins R, Armitage J, Parish S, et al. MRC/BHF Heart Protection Study of cholesterol-lowering with simvastatin in 5963 people with diabetes: a randomized placebo-controlled trial. *Lancet*. 2003;361:2005–2016.

15. Koponene H, Saari K, Savolainen M, et al. Weight gain and glucose and lipid metabolism disturbances during antipsychotic medication—a review. *Eur Arch Psychiatry Clin Neurosci*. 2002;252:294–298.

16. Meyer JM. Effects of atypical antipsychotics on weight and serum lipid levels. *J Clin Psychiatry*. 2001;62;40–41.

17. Ananth J, Parameswaran S, Gunatilake S. Side effects of atypical antipsychotic drugs. *Curr Pharmaceut Design*. 2004;10:2219–2229.

18. Lohr JB, Flynn K. Smoking and schizophrenia. *Schizophr Res*. 1992;8(2):93–102.

19. Hennekens CH, Hennekens AR, Hollar D, et al. Schizophrenia and increased risks of cardiovascular disease. *Am Heart J*. 2005;150:1115–1121.

20. de Leon J, Susce MT, Diaz FJ, et al. Variables associated with alcohol, drug, and daily smoking cessation in patients with severe mental illness. *J Clin Psychiatry*. 2005;66(11):1447–1455.

21. American Diabetes Association, American Psychiatric Association, American Association of Clinical Endocrinologists, and North American Association for the Study of Obesity. Consensus Development Conference on Antipsychotic Drugs and Obesity and Diabetes. *Obes Res.* 2004;12(2):362–368.
22. Mattock MB, Morrish NJ, Viberti G, et al. Prospective study of microalbuminuria as predictor of mortality in NIDDM. *Diabetes.* 1992;41(6);736–741.
23. Jablonowski K, Margolese HC, Chouinard G. Gabapentin-induced paradoxical exacerbation of psychosis in a patient with schizophrenia. *Can J Psychiatry.* 2002;47(10):975–976.
24. Tuomilehto J, Lindstrom J, Erikkson JG, et al. Prevention of type 2 diabetes mellitus by changes in lifestyle among subjects with impaired glucose tolerance. *New Engl J Med.* 2001;344(18):1343–1350.
25. Ratner RE. An update on the Diabetes Prevention Program. *Endocr Pract.* 2006;12(1):20–24.
26. Lindstrom J, Illane-Parikka P, Peltonen M, et al. Sustained reduction in the incidence of type 2 diabetes by lifestyle intervention: follow-up of the Finnish Diabetes Prevention Study. *Lancet.*2006;368(9548):1673–1679.
27. Tuomilehto J. Counterpoint: evidence-based prevention of type 2 diabetes: the power of lifestyle management. *Diabetes Care.* 2007;30(2):435–438.
28. Nathan DM, Buse JB, Davidson MB, et al. Management of hyperglycemia in type 2 diabetes: a consensus algorithm for the initiation and adjustment of therapy. *Diabetes Care.* 2006;29(8):1963–1972.
29. Cleveland JC, Meldrum DR, Cain BS, et al. Oral sulfonylurea hypoglycemic agents prevent ischemic preconditioning in human myocardium. *Circulation.* 1997;96:29–32.
30. UK Prospective Diabetes Study (UKPDS) Group. Effect of intensive blood-glucose control with metformin on complications in overweight patients with type 2 diabetes (UKPDS 34). *Lancet.* 1998;352:854–865.
31. Hanefeld M, Cagatay M, Petrowitsch T, et al. Acarbose reduces the risk for myocardial infarction in type 2 diabetic patients: meta-analysis of seven long-term studies. *Eur Heart J.* 2003;25(1):10–16.
32. Cavalot F, Petrelli A, Traversa M, et al. Postprandial blood glucose is a stronger predictor of cardiovascular events than fasting blood glucose in type 2 diabetes mellitus; particularly in women: lessons from the San Luigi Gonzaga Diabetes Study. *J Clin Endocrinol Metab.* 2006;91(3):813–819.
33. Nissen SE, Wolski K. Effect of rosiglitazone on the risk of myocardial infarction and death from cardiovascular causes. *New England Journal of Medicine.* 2007;356(24):2457–2471.
34. Grey A, Bolland M, Gamble G, et al. The peroxisome-proliferator-activated receptor-gamma agonist rosiglitazone decreases bone formation and bone mineral density in healthy postmenopausal women: A randomized, controlled trial. *Journal of Clinical Endocrinology & Metabolism.* 2007;92(4):1305–1310.
35. The DREAM (Diabetes REduction Assessment with ramipril and rosiglitazone Medication) Trial Investigators. Effect of rosiglitazone on the frequency of diabetes in patients with impaired glucose tolerance or impaired fasting glucose: a randomized controlled trial. *Lancet.* 2006;368:1096–1105.
36. Xu G, Stoffers DA, Habener JF, et al. Exendin-4 stimulates both beta-cell replication and neogenesis, resulting in increased beta-cell mass and improved glucose tolerance in diabetic rates. *Diabetes.* 1999;48(12):2270–2276.

37. Nasrallah HA, Newcomer JW. Atypical antipsychotics and metabolic dysregulation—evaluating the risk/benefit equation and improving the standard of care. *J Clin Psychopharmacol.* 2004;24(1):S7–S14.
38. Lacro JP, Dunn LB, Dolder CR, et al. Prevalence of and risk factors for medication nonadherence in patients with schizophrenia: a comprehensive review of recent literature. *J Clin Psychiatry,.*2002;63(10):892–909.

Patient Education Handouts

Mental Illness and Medications
How They Affect My Cardiovascular Health

Mental illness
- Symptoms of mental illness may decrease my interest in exercise and eating a healthy diet

Although medications help control mental illness, they may be associated with possible side effects such as:
- Weight gain
- High cholesterol
- High blood glucose, or diabetes

Medications associated with *weight gain*
- Antipsychotics
  - Clozapine, olanzapine, quetiapine, risperidone
- Antidepressants
  - Mirtazapine, paroxetine, amitriptyline
- Mood stabilizers
  - Divalproex sodium (Depakote), valproic acid, carbamazepine, lithium

Medications associated with *high cholesterol*
- Antipsychotics
  - Clozapine, olanzapine, quetiapine, risperidone
- Antidepressants
  - Mirtazapine

Medications associated with *high glucose* or *diabetes*
- Antipsychotics
  - Clozapine, olanzapine, quetiapine, risperidone
- Antidepressants
  - Amitriptyline, imipramine

For more information, talk with your psychiatrist, primary care doctor, endocrinologist (diabetes doctor), pharmacist, and dietician. They can help develop a management plan that is specific to you.

Created by: Jennifer A. Rosen, Pharm.D., BCPP, Donna A. Wirshing, M.D., and Cara F. Adamson Greene, Pharm.D.

What are the dangers associated with obesity, high cholesterol, and diabetes?

Dangers of *obesity*

- Diabetes
- Heart disease
- High blood pressure
- Cancer
- Sleep apnea (difficulty breathing while asleep)
- Osteoarthritis (wearing away of joints and cartilage)
- Poor self-image

Dangers of *high cholesterol*

- Atherosclerosis (narrowing of the blood vessels due to cholesterol deposits)
- Heart disease
- Pancreatitis (inflammation of the pancreas due to high triglycerides)
- Risk of stroke or heart attack

Dangers of *diabetes*

- Poor circulation
- Heart disease
- Risk of stroke or heart attack
- Nerve damage, nerve pain
- Loss of eyesight, blindness
- Risk of amputation
- Kidney damage or failure

Important: Do *not* stop taking your psychiatric medications if you experience any of the problems listed above. Talk with your doctor about ways to prevent or manage these problems.

Created by: Jennifer A. Rosen, Pharm.D., BCPP, Donna A. Wirshing, M.D., and Cara F. Adamson Greene, Pharm.D.

What can I do to maintain my health?

The *three key* components are:
- Diet
- Exercise
- Take your medications as directed by your doctor

Diet
- **Limit to no more than one serving per day:**
  - **High-sugar beverages** (avoid if you have diabetes)
    - Regular soda (1 can)
    - Fruit juices (1 cup)
  - **Sweets** (avoid if you have diabetes)
    - Pastries (2 × 2 square)
    - Cookies (1 to 2 small cookies)
    - Cakes (2 × 2 square)
    - Pies (1/8-piece pie)

- **Eat foods that will help you lose or maintain weight:**
  - **High-fiber foods** (they will keep you fuller longer)
    - Whole wheat bread
    - Oatmeal, cold oat cereals such as Cheerios
    - Beans, lentils
    - Fruits, vegetables
  - **Healthy snacks**
    - Vegetables
    - Fresh fruit
    - Low-fat cottage cheese
    - Graham crackers
    - Low-fat yogurt
    - Caffeine-free coffee or tea

Exercise
- Exercise for 30 to 45 minutes/day (talk to your doctor before starting an exercise program)
  - Cardiovascular: walking briskly, bicycling, swimming
  - Resistance training: using light weights or resistance bands

Medications
- Your doctor may prescribe medications to manage your cholesterol and glucose
- Take your medications as directed

Created by: Jennifer A. Rosen, Pharm.D., BCPP, Donna A. Wirshing, M.D., and Cara F. Adamson Greene, Pharm.D.

INDEX

Note: Page numbers followed by "f" refer to figures; page numbers followed by "t" refer to tables.

A

Acarbose, 119t
Addison disease, 2
Alpha-glucosidase inhibitors, 119t, 122
American Diabetes Association, screening
    recommendations, 112
Amputation, diabetes-related, 24, 25t
Amylin analogues, 123
Anorexiants, 101–102
Antidepressants. *See also specific drugs*
    body weight changes and, 52t
    glucose metabolism and, 52t
    monoamine oxidase inhibitors. *See*
        Monoamine oxidase inhibitors
    selective serotonin reuptake inhibitors.
        See Selective serotonin reuptake
        inhibitors
    tricyclic. *See* Tricyclic antidepressants
Antihypertensives, 113–114
Antipsychotics. *See also specific drugs*
    atypical/second-generation. *See*
        Atypical antipsychotics
    diabetes and, 58
    litigation concerning, 44–46
    side effects comparison, 73t
Aripiprazole
    body weight changes and, 60
    FDA review, 45–46
    side effects, vs. other antipsychotics,
        73t, 74t
Asparaginase, 77t
Aspirin therapy, 114
Atypical antidepressants, 54
Atypical antipsychotics. *See also specific
    drugs*
    advantages, 58
    adverse outcomes, 72t
    body weight changes and, 59–61,
        72t, 74t
    diabetes incidence and, 7, 58, 61–62
    dyslipidemia and, 70–71, 74t
    glucose metabolism and, 61–70, 74t, 77t
    litigation concerning, 44–46

mechanisms of action, 58–59
    metabolic monitoring recommenda-
        tions, 69–70, 70t, 115
    metabolic syndrome and, 59
    side effects, 58–59, 73t, 74t
Autism, risperidone for, 61

B

Bariatric surgery, 101
Bed days, 16
Benzodiazepines, 78
Beta adrenergic blockers, 77t
Beta agonists, 77t
Biguanides, 118t, 122
Bipolar illness
    diabetes in, 7–11, 89
    polycystic ovary syndrome and, 9–11
Blood glucose monitoring, 98–99, 126
Blood pressure, venlafaxine and, 54.
    See also Hypertension
Body mass index (BMI), 86. *See also*
    Obesity
Body weight changes
    antidepressants and, 50t, 53–57
    antipsychotics and, 59–61, 72–74t
    carbamazepine and, 75
    lamotrigine and, 76
    lithium and, 74–75
    management. *See* Body weight
        management
    patterns, health risks and, 59–60
    valproate and, 76
Body weight management
    behavioral therapy, 99–100
    benefits, 38
    challenges in the mentally ill, 88–90
    exercise, 99
    nutritional interventions
        basic concepts, 103–105
        blood sugar monitoring, 98–99
        caloric distribution recommenda-
            tions, 94–95

135

screening and diagnosis, 111–112
treatment
blood glucose monitoring in, 126
body weight management. *See* Body
weight management
challenges in mental illness, 126–127
exercise, 125–126
goals, 112–114
lifestyle modification, 117
nonglycemic goals, 126
pharmacologic
guidelines for initiation, 124–125
insulin regimens, 120–122t,
123–124
oral hypoglycemic agents,
118–119t, 122–123
smoking cessation, 114, 126
type 1
depression and, 3–4
pathophysiology, 111
retinopathy in, 116
schizophrenia and, 6
type 2
bipolar illness and, 8–9
depression and, 4
pathophysiology, 111
retinopathy in, 116
schizophrenia and, 6
Diabetes Food Guide Pyramid, 95, 95f
Diabetic nephropathy
costs, 26–27, 28t
management, 115–116
Diabetic retinopathy, 116
Diazoxide, 77t
Didanosine, 77t
Disability, diabetes-related, 17, 18t
Diuretics, 77t
Divalproex sodium. *See* Valproate
Duloxetine, 53–54
Dyslipidemia
atypical antipsychotics and, 70–71,
72–74t
mirtazapine and, 55–56
treatment goals in diabetics, 114

E
EMSAM. *See* Selegiline
Encainide, 77t
End-stage renal failure, diabetes-related

costs, 26–27, 28t
prevention, 115–116
Exchange lists, for meal planning,
96–97, 97t
Exercise, in diabetes, 99

F
Fat, 104
Fiber, 104–105
Fluoxetine, 52t, 57
Foot ulcers, diabetes-related. *See* Lower-
extremity ulcers, diabetes-
related

G
Gastric bypass surgery, 101
Glimepiride, 118t
Glipizide, 118t, 122
GLP-1 analogues, 123
Glucocorticoid dysfunction, 2
Glucose metabolism
antidepressants and, 52t, 53–57
atypical antipsychotics and, 61–70,
67–68t
drugs affecting, 49, 50t, 51t, 77
lithium and, 75
in schizophrenia, 7
valproate and, 76
Glulisine, 120t
Glyburide, 118t, 122
Glycemic targets, 113

H
Haloperidol, 73t
Health care expenditures, U.S., diabetes
and, 15
Hyperglycemia, 111. *See also* Glucose
metabolism
Hypertension, 38, 113–114
Hypertriglyceridemia. *See* Dyslipidemia
Hypoglycemia, drugs associated with, 51t

I
Imipramine, 77t
Impaired fasting glucose, 111
Impaired glucose tolerance, 111